Fibromyalgia
MANAGING THE PAIN
SECOND EDITION

Mark J. Pellegrino, M.D.

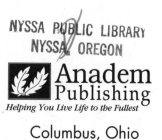
Anadem
Publishing
Helping You Live Life to the Fullest

Columbus, Ohio

FIBROMYALGIA
MANAGING THE PAIN
SECOND EDITION

Anadem Publishing, Inc.
Columbus, Ohio 43214
614 • 262 • 2539
800 • 633 • 0055
http://www.anadem.com

Printed in the U.S.A.
ISBN 1-890018-10-4

The material in *Fibromyalgia: Managing the Pain, Second Edition* is
presented for informational purposes only. It is not meant to be a substitute for proper medical care by your doctor. You need to consult
with your doctor for diagnosis and treatment.

Acknowledgements

This book is dedicated to my fibromyalgia patients, especially those who have shared their hearts and souls to the support group.

A special thanks to:

George W. Waylonis, M.D. for diagnosing my fibromyalgia, and whose teaching, support and encouragement have helped inspire me to research and treat people with fibromyalgia. Dr. Waylonis and I worked together on fibromyalgia research projects supported by the Fibromyalgia Association of Central Ohio.

Karol Noftsinger for her help in preparing this book.

Numerous investigators around the world have contributed to research and understanding of fibromyalgia. I have tried to combine the important research findings along with my personal and professional experience into this book.

Table of Contents

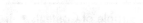

Introduction

Fibromyalgia is a common painful condition of soft tissues, mainly muscles, which causes widespread pain, stiffness, fatigue and poor sleep, among other symptoms.

I have fibromyalgia and understand how this condition affects your everyday life because of persistent pain. Ever since I was diagnosed with this condition, I have sought to learn as much as I can by conducting research projects, attending international symposiums, and reading the latest medical literature. I have also learned much from the many patients with fibromyalgia that I treat in my private practice, and I have the unique opportunity of bridging both my personal and professional interests in this condition.

Years ago, I wrote a detailed handout to give to my newly diagnosed fibromyalgia patients. Periodically I would update the handout as new information was learned. During a recent revision, many of my patients encouraged me to expand on my handout and develop this book.

The purposes of this book are to provide you with updated, comprehensive and understandable information about fibromyalgia and to share some of my personal experiences in dealing with this condition. Hopefully, you will develop a good understanding of fibromyalgia and learn positive strategies for successfully coping with your painful condition.

Although this book contains detailed information about fibromyalgia, it is not meant to be a substitute for proper medical care by your doctor. All the contents in this book are for information purposes only and you need to consult with your doctor for diagnosis and treatment.

1

History

Fibromyalgia has been around for a long time, even though we have only recently begun to better understand and diagnose this condition. In 1904, the medical literature first described the condition of "fibrositis" as a cause of low back pain. Initial medical investigators at the turn of the century reported that they had seen, under a microscope, inflamed areas in the fibrous tissue or fascia that surrounds muscles and binds them together. Hence the name fibrositis, which implied that the cause of the pain was a fibrous tissue inflammation. We now know this is not the case. With the advent of more sophisticated microscopes and more carefully designed research studies, medical investigators have shown that there is no actual inflammation in the muscle or connective tissue of these patients.

Because the original opinion that an inflammation existed was wrong, many doctors concluded, falsely, that fibrositis was not even a legitimate condition, and that the patients' symptoms were "all in their head." In fact, many physicians used the term "psychogenic rheumatism" to describe fibrositis.

In the past 15 years, there has been a renewed interest in studying this condition. The term "fibromyalgia" (fibro-fiber, my-muscle, algia-pain) has gradually replaced "fibrositis" as the name of choice because fibrositis incorrectly implies inflammation. Fibrositis and fibromyalgia both mean the same thing.

In 1981, Dr. Yunus described criteria which were used as a standard to objectively diagnose patients with fibromyalgia. A virtual explosion of research has occurred in the past decade. There have been descriptions of a condition called myofascial pain syndrome, characterized by regional muscle pain and tender points that may be a localized version of the generalized fibromyalgia. Much has been published on both of these conditions.

In 1989, investigators worldwide convened in Minneapolis, Minnesota for the first International

> Fibromyalgia is now recognized as a distinct medical condition with characteristic findings.

Myofascial Pain and Fibromyalgia symposium to present research and share knowledge. In 1990, the American College of Rheumatology devised updated fibromyalgia criteria based on a multi-regional study. In 1992, the second International Myofascial Pain and Fibromyalgia symposium was held in Copenhagen, Denmark. These symposiums have attracted hundreds of medical professionals throughout the world interested in fibromyalgia. In 1995, the Third International Myofascial Pain and Fibromyalgia Symposium was held in San Antonio, Texas with the emphasis on pathologic mechanisms. The Fourth International Symposium is planned for 1998 in Italy.

Fibromyalgia is now recognized as a distinct medical condition with characteristic findings.

Fibromyalgia is a syndrome of widespread pain involving mainly muscle, but also tendons (which hold muscles to bone), ligaments (which hold bones together), bursa (fluid-filled sacs that decrease the friction over the joints) and joints. The pain is generalized usually, but distinct areas of tenderness in specific locations are characteristic. Tenderness in one spot is referred to as a tender point. If pressing on the tender point causes pain to spread or radiate to another area, this spot is called a trigger point. The 1990 American College of Rheumatology criteria identify 18 body locations, of which at least 11 must be tender in order to make the diagnosis of fibromyalgia. I will discuss these criteria further in Chapter 9.

2

Fibromyalgia: What It Is

"When a man begins to understand himself, he begins to live."

– Norvin G. McGranahan

The muscle pain fluctuates and is often aggravated by various physical, environmental and emotional factors. In addition to causing pain, fibromyalgia causes stiffness (especially in the morning), fatigue, numbness, feeling of weakness, swelling, cold intolerance, poor sleep and dry eyes. Various conditions have been linked with fibromyalgia, including tension and migraine headaches, irritable bowel syndrome, TMJ dysfunction, irritable bladder, depression and chronic fatigue syndrome.

Fibromyalgia can be classified into several types:

1. **Primary fibromyalgia.** This type is the most common. It occurs in the absence of an underlying rheumatologic disease such as rheumatoid arthritis or lupus. Hereditary predisposition may play a major role in who develops this type of fibromyalgia.

2. **Secondary (or reactive) fibromyalgia.** This occurs in the presence of an underlying disease such as rheumatoid arthritis, lupus, hypothyroidism, cancer or AIDS. A special category of secondary fibromyalgia is called posttraumatic fibromyalgia, which is commonly seen following a trauma such as a motor vehicle accident.

> Fibromyalgia is a syndrome of widespread pain involving mainly muscle, but also tendons, ligaments, bursa, and joints.

3. **Concomitant fibromyalgia.** This is thought to occur along with another condition such as osteoarthritis or scoliosis, with no clear relationship.

4. **Myofascial pain syndrome.** Some individuals believe this is a regional or localized form of fibromyalgia, and others consider it a separate entity altogether. Muscle trauma commonly causes this condition, which may develop into a more generalized state. The key findings in myofascial pain syndrome are tender points and trigger points.

Fibromyalgia used to be called by various other names, including fibrositis, myofibrositis, fibromyositis, nonrestorative sleep disorder, nonarticular rheumatism, myofascial pain syndrome, and tension myalgia. Today, fibromyalgia is considered the medically correct term to describe this painful condition.

Fibromyalgia is not a tumor. It is not a deforming arthritis such as rheumatoid arthritis. It is not a paralyzing or progressive neurologic disorder like multiple sclerosis or Lou Gehrig's disease. It is not a ruptured disk or a pinched nerve, even though your symptoms may resemble those caused by a pinched nerve.

Fibromyalgia is not even classified as a disease, but rather as a syndrome. This is not to say that the pain is not a problem, because it can cause functional limitations varying from mild to incapacitating.

In its technical sense, the word disease implies a destructive, irreversible, progressive or abnormal process that causes alteration of body tissues and can be isolated and often treated. A syndrome is usually a name ascribed to a cluster of symptoms, often symptoms that do not have a single pathologic abnormality. Not all terminology in medicine is "grammatically" correct, in that some syndromes are really diseases, such as carpal tunnel syndrome or Down's syndrome, and some diseases are really syndromes, such as Raynaud's disease.

Because fibromyalgia causes symptoms resembling those of a pinched nerve or arthritis, patients often mistake it for a serious disease. Once I understood that my fibromyalgia was not going to paralyze me, deform me or act like a cancer, I became less frightened of the condition. Even though the pain is very real and very THERE, I feel my understanding of fibromyalgia allows me to cope with it better.

In your fight against fibromyalgia, I believe over half the battle is won once you begin to understand the condition.

3

Fibromyalgia: What It Is Not

"If you worry about what might be, and wonder what might have been, you will ignore what is."

– Unknown

Anyone can get fibromyalgia, but it is diagnosed about seven times more in women than men. Children can also have fibromyalgia, although the condition usually first causes symptoms between ages 25 and 45. Usually, the symptoms have been present for years even though the diagnosis may not have been made until after age 50. Worldwide, about 5% of the population has this condition, so it is very common, and it affects millions and millions of people. In order to "officially" have fibromyalgia, one must be seen by a physician. Many people out there have fibromyalgia who have yet to see a physician and be officially diagnosed.

4

Fibromyalgia: Who Gets It

"None of us can be free of conflict and woe. Even the greatest men have had to accept disappointments as their daily bread."

– Bernard M. Baruch

The key complaint with fibromyalgia is pain. Many of my patients say the primary problem is, "I hurt all over." This pain may be described as a constant ache, nag or throbbing. Typical pain locations include the head, neck, shoulders (especially between the shoulder blades), low back and hip muscles. Chest pain can also be a problem, especially in large-busted women. Certain areas may cause sharp, stabbing pain. The patient can often point to the exact areas of pain and note that these particular areas are very sensitive to touch.

About half the time, there is no clear reason why the pain occurs; that is, there has been no specific illness or trauma: usually the pain begins in one location, such as the shoulder, but over time it begins to involve more and more other areas until it is no longer localized, but rather generalized throughout the body.

In about half the patients, some type of event, either an injury such as a whiplash or a viral illness such as mononucleosis, precipitated the fibromyalgia condition. In these people, the pain started quickly after the event and never disappeared.

The pain may wander to different sites; the low back may be sore one day and then the next day it is the neck that hurts. These wandering symptoms may lead you to think you are going crazy! I was convinced there could be no possible physical condition that would cause wandering pain and that therefore I must be nuts. Once I learned that fibromyalgia indeed causes wandering pain, I knew that I wasn't as completely crazy as I thought.

The muscles are not the only sore areas. Other soft tissues, such as the ligaments, tendons and bursa, can be sore. Bursitis and tendonitis, especially in the shoulder, elbow and hip, are common in patients with fibromyalgia. Another common area of pain is in the sternum, or breast plate, where the ribs attach. This is called costochondritis and can mimic heart pain, but there is nothing wrong with the heart.

5

Fibromyalgia Complaints

"You will suffer and you will hurt. You will have joy and you will have peace."

– Alison Cheek

Symptoms of Fibromyalgia	
Muscle pain	Poor Sleep
Fatigue	Cold Intolerance
Stiffness	Headaches
Numbness	Joint Pain
Weakness	Tendinitis
Swelling	Tingling

Atypical chest wall pain is frightening to people, especially if it is a new area of pain in fibromyalgia. The heart muscle is not affected by fibromyalgia, however.

Joint pain and stiffness are also usually present. They are mostly related to pain at the muscle and tendon insertions into the joint area, and not to actual joint pathology or inflammation. The skin is also described as extremely sensitive and painful in many patients with fibromyalgia.

There may be tingling, numbness, swelling, or feelings of heat or cold with fibromyalgia. These abnormal sensations are called paresthesias. The pain and paresthesias may radiate or travel to different locations. For example, painful muscle areas in the upper back may cause the arms to become painful and tingling, even though there is no problem, per se, in the arm.

Poor sleep is a hallmark in nearly all patients with fibromyalgia. Patients report that the quality of their sleep is poor. Even though they may sleep for eight hours, and when they awaken in the morning they do not feel well rested. Sleep may be characterized by frequent awakening, especially in the early morning hours, and lack of deep, sound sleep.

I do not have difficulty falling asleep, but I usually wake up around 4 a.m. I feel "ready to go" at that time, but I realize it is too early to get up. So I lay in bed frequently glancing at the clock, never falling back into a deep sleep. Once it is finally time to get up, I feel exhausted and with great effort, I must drag myself out of bed.

This disturbed and nonrestorative sleep pattern is typical of patients with fibromyalgia. Sleep studies using EEG monitors to measure brain waves of sleeping individuals have found that there is an abnormality in the deep sleep stage. This lack of deep sleep accounts for the feeling that our sleep was nonrestorative or that "our battery did not get recharged" during the night.

Next to pain, general fatigue is the major complaint with fibromyalgia. The poor sleep certainly contributes to this problem, but patients with fibromyalgia will often indicate that they have no energy whatsoever, that they cannot get motivated to do various projects, and that they would rather lie down and go to sleep.

Most patients report morning stiffness, usually lasting a few hours. They feel somewhat looser and better during the late morning to early evening, then have more pain again in the evening. Most people would say the worst time of the day is in the morning. Instead of waking up refreshed and pain-free, we wake up tired, stiff and sore! Once we get going, our muscles loosen up within a few hours, and we are fairly limber, until later in the day. This morning stiffness may be particularly bad the day after doing strenuous or unusual activities.

> Most people would say the worst time of the day is in the morning. Instead of waking up refreshed and pain-free, we wake up tired, stiff and sore!

Fibromyalgia symptoms can be modulated by certain factors. That is, there are very specific factors that cause our symptoms to either worsen or improve. Some factors can precipitate a full-blown flare-up. These modulating factors fall into several categories:

Physical Factors

Certain physical activities can cause flare-ups in fibromyalgia symptoms. Performing a strenuous activity, such as moving furniture or playing hours of volleyball on a Sunday afternoon, can aggravate the symptoms and set up a rather vicious cycle of increased pain, even though you have stopped the activity. Post-exercise pain is common even with "ordinary" exercise. Like too much activity, too little activity can also aggravate the symptoms.

I learned firsthand how decreased physical activity could cause worsening of my fibromyalgia. During my last year of residency, I became involved in so many projects that I was unable to continue my exercise program on a regular basis. Gradually, I noticed that my low back became more uncomfortable and was easily "twisted." It got to the point where just bending over to pick up a Kleenex caused sharp, knife-like pains in my back that lasted for a few days before gradually fading. Once I realized what was happening, I resumed my exercise program and within a short period, my symptoms improved and my back became "stable" again. I learned that never again could I afford to neglect my exercises because I (especially my back) would pay the price.

Certain positions that require sustained isometric muscle contraction, such as holding our arms out in front of us for a long time, are not tolerated well by people with fibromyalgia. Our muscles, especially the ones in the shoulders, do not like sustained contraction to hold our arms in one place, and they communicate this to us by PAIN: pain in the neck, shoulders and back. Every day activities requiring this positioning include typing, assembly line work, putting things on shelves, driving, playing the piano, and many more.

6

Modulating Factors in Fibromyalgia

"Everyday...life confronts us with new problems to be solved which force us to adjust our old programs accordingly."

– Dr. Ann Faraday

<table>
<tr><td>

Modulating Factors in Fibromyalgia

Physical

Environmental

Psychosocial

Spontaneous

</td></tr>
</table>

As I look back to my childhood, I can remember that changing a ceiling light bulb used to cause my arm to feel like all the energy drained out of it. I would have to drop my arm down and wait a few minutes for the aching to subside and the "strength" to return before I could finish changing the bulb. Only in the past few years did I finally understand that my fibromyalgia caused this weakness, even at a young age.

The more tired we are and the longer we maintain these activities, the more discomfort we have. Recognizing and avoiding or modifying these aggravating conditions are crucial to the control of the symptoms.

Most people will experience an increase in their symptoms when they have a viral infection or flu syndrome, or even after getting a flu vaccine. Some women note a flare-up of their symptoms just before their period starts. This may be related to increased muscle swelling during the fluid-retention stage of their menstrual cycle. In fact, the common premenstrual syndrome (PMS) is often more severe in women with fibromyalgia.

Environmental Factors

Patients with fibromyalgia are very sensitive to weather changes, especially cold, damp conditions and cold drafts. One of my major enemies is the cold air-conditioner draft on the back of my neck, which will absolutely exacerbate my neck and shoulder pain. Even if we are completely relaxed and enjoying ourselves, a cold draft on exposed skin overlying tender muscle areas can cause an automatic reflexive reaction which sends a signal to the muscles and causes muscle pain. In patients with fibromyalgia, the skin is very sensitive, especially to cold air. Likewise, cold water is bad for patients with fibromyalgia, and they do not do well in pools where the water temperature is lower than skin temperature.

Weather changes can also cause fibromyalgia symptoms to increase, especially if it is cold or damp. It appears that muscles act like barometers to the weather. When it is colder and damper, perhaps our muscles absorb more moisture or are more swollen or sensitive, which may cause the increased pain. Whatever the reason, patients with fibromyalgia do best in warm, dry regions or during warmer, dryer seasons. I do not advocate that all fibromyalgia patients move to Arizona, but a periodic vacation there, especially during winter, may be helpful!

> I learned that never again could I afford to neglect my exercises because... I would pay the price.

Psychosocial Factors

People with fibromyalgia seem to have a certain type of personality, known as the fibromyalgia personality. Individuals tend to be compulsive, highly organized, perfectionistic, time-oriented, and anxious. We like to do things ourselves because we know it will get done exactly the way we want. We cannot trust others to get the job done "right," so we end up doing most everything ourselves. It really bothers us when others do not respect details and time as we do.

Because we are so compulsive, we are not satisfied with just getting a job done; we want it to be the best job ever done. Consequently, no matter what we do, whether at work or home, we are always putting pressure on ourselves to do the best that we can. That sets us up for emotional stress, which can cause our muscles to tense up. I believe that even if we change our job to testing recliner chairs, we would still be stressed out because we would want to be the best recliner chair testers ever!

Without a doubt, emotional stress plays a major role in fibromyalgia flare-ups, but everyday emotional stress is not felt to be the cause of fibromyalgia. Some people have traced the onset of their fibromyalgia to an unusual "catastrophic" stressful period in their life. Stress is a part of life, but our high levels of expectation seem to make usual stressors more bothersome. If things do not go well, if

> Emotional stress plays a major role in fibromyalgia flare-ups, but emotional stress is not felt to be the cause of fibromyalgia.

deadlines are not met, if unexpected circumstances arise, we feel the stress more. This stress will increase fibromyalgia symptoms.

Persons with fibromyalgia have more anxiety and depression than those without this condition, and they will report more functional disability in their everyday life activities compared to someone who does not have this condition. It is important that stressors be identified and dealt with to minimize fibromyalgia flare-ups and potential psychosocial complications.

Spontaneous Factors

Perhaps the most common cause of fibromyalgia flare-ups is "unknown" cause. Frequently, a fibromyalgia flare-up is unrelated to any physical, environmental or psychosocial factor; the pain just spontaneously increases with no traceable offending factor. When this happens, it is frustrating because a person may be doing all the "right" things, yet still experiences a flare-up beyond his or her control.

Many other conditions are frequently seen with fibromyalgia. These conditions themselves are commonly present without fibromyalgia, but are seen frequently enough with fibromyalgia that there may be an overlapping link. The following conditions have been reported or observed to be commonly associated with fibromyalgia.

1. **Allergies**. The majority of patients with fibromyalgia have some history of allergies, either themselves or family members. The offending allergenic substance may be any type of environmental allergen, such as dust or pollen. It may be a medication. Sensitivity to smells is common and may have an allergic mechanism. We are not certain what is the specific relationship between allergies and fibromyalgia, but it may reflect involvement of the immune system and sympathetic nerves.

2. **Anxiety disorder and panic attacks**. Many people with fibromyalgia experience episodes of extreme anxiety and near-panic. They may feel their heart racing, feel their chest become tight and find it difficult to get their breath. There may be a feeling of impending doom. An extreme sensitivity to adrenaline or oversensitive sympathetic nervous system may be a cause of this associated condition.

3. **Concentration and memory problems**. Studies have not shown any true pathology in one's thinking and memory with fibromyalgia. However, many people with fibromyalgia report forgetfulness, absentmindedness, confusion, and a feeling of being in a fog. They become very frustrated and concerned by these symptoms. The chronic pain may divert our attention that would otherwise be used to initiate the process of forming memory. Low serotonin level, mental fatigue, and altered brain neurologic activity probably contribute to this problem. When consciously attending to a specific task or specific

7

Conditions Seen with Fibromyalgia

"Difficulties are meant to rouse, not to discourage. The human spirit is to grow strong by conflict."

– William Ellery Channing

information, people with fibromyalgia demonstrate normal learning and memory, but do so more slowly than persons without fibromyalgia.

I used to think I was losing my memory when I noticed more frequent misplacing keys, and pens, and forgetting names and appointments. After I understood that my memory was fine, but my attention was being diverted to monitoring pain and not integrating new information into my memory banks, I became less concerned. I write everything in my daily calendar to avoid "forgetting" important things. Now, if I could only remember to look at my calendar each day!

4. **Depression**. Depression is commonly seen in conditions that cause chronic pain, including fibromyalgia. Usual symptoms of depression include low self esteem, feeling of helplessness, thoughts of suicide, poor appetite, frequent crying spells and more. People with fibromyalgia who become clinically depressed need treatment of both the depression and the fibromyalgia to get well again.

5. **Dry eyes syndrome**. Up to a third of patients with fibromyalgia report dry eyes. Many have to use eye drops to prevent painful reddened eyes.

6. **Headaches: tension, migraine, and combination**. Tension headaches are also called muscle contraction headaches, which usually begin at the base of the neck and extend upward to the temples, often forming what is described as a band-like, squeezing headache. Migraine headaches are vascular headaches in which some event triggers the blood vessels to the brain to constrict and then dilate, leading to a severe headache, nausea, vomiting, eye pain and other symptoms. Many people have headaches which have both tension and migraine features.

7. **Irritable bladder**. The individual may feel like he or she has a bladder infection, with frequent painful urination, but urine tests do not reveal any evidence of infection.

8. **Irritable bowel syndrome or spastic colon**. Nearly half of patients with fibromyalgia have frequent bowel cramping, diarrhea, and constipation.

> People with fibromyalgia who become clinically depressed need treatment of both the depression and the fibromyalgia to get well again.

9. **Mitral valve prolapse (MVP)**. MVP is a condition where one of the heart valves, the mitral valve, bulges excessively during the heartbeat. It can be diagnosed by listening with a stethoscope for the characteristic click-murmur, or it can be detected with a soundwave test called an echocardiogram. This condition can cause problems such as abnormal heart rhythm, but rarely so. In fact, most cardiologists feel that MVP is a benign condition that does not mean a bad heart disease is present. I conducted a study at The Ohio State University that showed that the majority of people with fibromyalgia also have MVP. Since the mitral valve is mostly connective tissue, it is possible that fibromyalgia affects connective tissue other than the muscles, tendons and ligaments.

10. **Restless leg syndrome and nocturnal myoclonus**. These related conditions are most prominent at night. Restless leg syndrome causes leg cramps, especially in the calves, and an intense feeling of restlessness in the leg, that is not relieved until the individual moves the leg, as in walking around. Nocturnal myoclonus is involuntary jerking that occurs during sleep. A neurologic mechanism, perhaps signals that don't get "turned off," may be responsible for both of these similar conditions.

11. **Raynaud's phenomenon**. This is characterized by intermittent attacks of white or blue discolorations of the fingers or toes. Cold or stress usually brings on these vascular changes.

> Many physicians believe chronic fatigue syndrome and fibromyalgia are actually the same thing.

12. **Scoliosis**. Curvature of the spine commonly develops in teenage girls for no apparent reason. Scoliosis is also seen in a number of neuromuscular diseases. I have observed a number of patients who have scoliosis and fibromyalgia.

13. **Temporomandibular joint dysfunction (TMJ dysfunction)**. This condition is characterized predominantly by painful jaws. Other symptoms of TMJ dysfunction include headaches, ringing in ears, face numbness and dizziness. This painful condition is treated by dental specialists.

14. **Chronic fatigue syndrome**. Many physicians believe chronic fatigue syndrome and fibromyalgia are actually the same thing. Chronic fatigue syndrome causes fatigue and pain, and it may be triggered by a virus. It is also associated with mild fever, sore throat, and swollen, painful lymph nodes, but severe fatigue and muscle pains are the predominant complaints.

15. **Gynecological conditions**. Several female conditions are commonly seen together with fibromyalgia. These include dysmenorrhea (painful menstrual cramping), vulvodynia (painful vaginal area), fibrocystic breast disease (painful breast cysts), and endometriosis (painful uterine tissue growths). Hormonal changes in women with fibromyalgia probably account for these conditions.

Various factors can lead to fibromyalgia, but the exact mechanism by which fibromyalgia develops is unknown. We have many theories now and I believe that ongoing research will soon lead to the exact mechanism of fibromyalgia – the "magic bullet." The following are various factors which may be important in helping us ultimately understand exactly how fibromyalgia develops.

8

Causes of Fibromyalgia

"We do not know one-millionth of one percent about anything."

– Thomas Edison

1. **Genetics**. Fibromyalgia may be an inherited condition that has an inactive stage. A research project that I undertook a few years ago showed that fibromyalgia may be inherited as an autosomal dominant condition. This means that if a parent has fibromyalgia, then half of her children have the potential to develop fibromyalgia also. Fibromyalgia can take years to fully develop, even though the genes may be there since birth, and it may skip generations. Several studies have supported the hereditary tendency of fibromyalgia.

   An interesting example occurred in twin girls who developed fibromyalgia symptoms within a few months of each other, even though they lived in different cities and were unaware of the other's condition. Often, children of a parent who has fibromyalgia will have commonly associated conditions, such as restless leg syndrome or localized chronic muscle pain, or unusual "growing pains," which alone are not indicative of fibromyalgia, but may signal that fibromyalgia syndrome will eventually develop.

2. **Trauma**. Trauma is a well-known cause of muscle pain. Many people never experience any problems with painful muscles until after some type of injury, such as an automobile accident or a job injury. Normally, such injuries completely heal within a few weeks, but in some people the injured muscles become chronically painful, even though the acute muscle injury has subsided. Posttraumatic fibromyalgia is detailed in Chapter 28.

> ## Possible Causes of Fibromyalgia
>
> Genetic
>
> Trauma
>
> Infections
>
> Muscle Physiology Problem
>
> Neurologic Mechanism
>
> Neurotransmitter Abnormality
>
> Abnormal Sleep Pattern
>
> Endocrine Abnormality
>
> Autoimmune Mechanism
>
> Structural Muscle Change
>
> Allergic Factors

3. **Infections**. Many times a viral infection, such as mononucleosis or a flu syndrome, can precipitate fibromyalgia. Chronic fatigue syndrome has been mentioned as a commonly associated condition that may have an infectious origin. As I've indicated earlier, many physicians believe that chronic fatigue syndrome and fibromyalgia are the same thing. A genetic susceptibility to certain chronic viral disorders may exist that causes an individual to develop fibromyalgia after exposure to a particular virus, or the particular virus may damage or activate certain neurologic functions of the body and lead to fibromyalgia. The virus may cause a chronic "low-grade" infection, or the virus may just leave its "mark" and disappear.

4. **Muscle physiology problem**. Decreased oxygen supply to muscles with fibromyalgia may account for some of the pain mechanism. Some studies have shown a lower concentration of energy-rich proteins and a lower concentration of oxygen in muscles with fibromyalgia. When the muscles contract, less energy is available to sustain these contractions. There may be impaired blood circulation to the muscles, causing less oxygen availability for the muscles during contractions. The combination of decreased oxygen and energy causes early muscle fatigue and less efficient contractions, leading to muscle pain. These factors may cause increased tension or spasms within the muscles, which also contribute to the pain and may account for the feeling of constant muscle tightness or stiffness. Muscle action is determined by nerves and hormones. Whether the muscles are the primary problem, or whether they simply do what the nerves and hormones tell them to do (i.e.–hurt!) remains to be determined. Even though muscle pain is the main complaint, the main "problem" may lie outside the muscles.

Interestingly, tissues other than muscles have been found to have lower oxygen concentrations in patients with fibromyalgia. This supports the notion that fibromyalgia involves more than just muscle tissue.

> One of the hallmarks of fibromyalgia is nonrestorative sleep...this may contribute to the muscle pain and fatigue.

5. **Neurologic mechanism**. People with fibromyalgia may have an altered neurologic mechanism that accounts for some component of their pain. There are probably both peripheral mechanisms, changes within the nerves and muscles themselves, and central mechanisms,or changes within the brain and spinal cord, that lead to pain in fibromyalgia. The pain threshold is lower in fibromyalgia, particularly in the tender areas, and this may lead to a hypersensitive central nervous system response to pain. Reverberating or continuous neurologic pain circuits maybe activated that act like short circuits to cause chronic pain. Studies have shown differences in the brain in patients with fibromyalgia, including the limbic systems and hypothalamus which control the neuroendocrine and emotional responses to pain. Sex differences are also present in the brain.

Many feel that the sympathetic (or autonomic) nervous system is the key to fibromyalgia pathology. These small nerves are responsible for the physiologic controls of many body functions, including heart rate, skin temperature, sweating, swelling and pain.

Fibromyalgia patients have a dysfunctional sympathetic nervous system. Numerous symptoms attributed to this dysfunction include dizziness, lightheadedness, near fainting spells, night sweats, cold hands and feet, heart palpitations, anxiety, swelling, numbness, tingling, and more.

Tilt table testing can measure this sympathetic nerve dysfunction in fibromyalgia patients. Changes occur in the blood pressure and pulse when a fibromyalgia patient goes from a lying

> People with severe problems with dry eyes may have an autoimmune subtype of fibromyalgia.

down position to an upright tilted position. The blood pressure drops if the sympathetic nerves are unable to quickly adjust to the gravity forces on the body. Further research may reveal the sympathetic nervous system to be the "main" flaw in fibromyalgia.

6. **Neurotransmitter abnormalities**. Perhaps closely linked with neurologic factors are the neurotransmitters, which may be lacking or deficient in patients with fibromyalgia. Neurotransmitters are small proteins that activate nerve signals. Two particular compounds, found in abnormal concentrations in patients with fibromyalgia include substance P (higher than normal) and serotonin (lower than normal). These two neurotransmitters are important components in the altered pain mechanism of fibromyalgia patients.

7. **Endocrine (hormonal) abnormalities** Numerous hormones are felt to influence the fibromyalgia mechanisms. Decreased thyroid hormone and possibly decreased growth hormone may have an important role in causing fibromyalgia. Recent studies have shown that a product of growth hormone, called somatomedin C, is found in lower concentrations in patients with fibromyalgia. Estrogen may influence muscle pain in women through various mechanisms: lowering pain threshold, blocking the body's pain relieving pathways, and promoting brain pathways. Since women with fibromyalgia far outnumber men, we need to look closely at the estrogen role in causing fibromyalgia.

Endocrine and neurotransmitter abnormalities are closely linked and neuroendocrine mechanisms probably play important roles in fibromyalgia pathology.

8. **Abnormal sleep patterns**. One of the hallmarks of fibromyalgia is nonrestorative sleep, in which patients describe a feeling of nonrestful sleep even though they may be sleeping for eight hours. A specific EEG abnormality, known as alpha-delta sleep, is found in the majority of patients with fibromyalgia. With fibromyalgia, one is not able to obtain a normal deep sleep, and this may contribute to the muscle pain and fatigue.

> Some types of fibromyalgia are more like "normal" and other types are more like "disease."

9. **Autoimmune mechanism**. The body's immune system, for various reasons, can start to recognize some of the proteins as foreign. The body's defense mechanism actually starts attacking its own protein and, if severe enough, can cause serious illness. This happens in certain types of arthritis and connective tissue disease. A virus can trigger autoimmune-like changes. Chronic viral symptoms and autoimmune-type symptoms are very similar and may be caused by an overreactive immune system that follows certain viral infections.

In some people with fibromyalgia, however, the autoimmune mechanism appears to be very low grade because, as we know, it is not destructive or deforming like serious autoimmune diseases. More investigation needs to be done to clarify the autoimmune factor and determine whether it is a mechanism in all of fibromyalgia or just a certain subtype of fibromyalgia. People with severe problems with dry eyes may have an autoimmune subtype of fibromyalgia.

10. **Structural muscle changes**. Sophisticated microscopes have revealed some apparent structural abnormalities in fibromyalgia muscles. Investigators have noticed peculiar changes in the muscle fibers that resemble rippled and rubberband notches. It is not known whether these changes represent true abnormalities or are variants of normal. Other investigators have not found these types of changes, so

we are not sure if true, consistent structural changes exist in the fibromyalgia muscles.

11. **Allergic factors**. Some researchers have found increased histamine response, or allergic response, in the muscles and skin, which may account for swelling and redness changes seen in many individuals. There may be a muscle allergy in response to some type of protein or dietary substance. If there is indeed an allergic mechanism, it is likely to be closely linked with the autoimmune and sympathetic nervous systems.

I believe that fibromyalgia is a syndrome that falls in between the high normal and low disease categories. Individuals with this condition have a muscle make-up that may not be quite normal, even though the muscles function normally (except they hurt). But on the other hand, it is not a true disease, even though it has some features of a "low grade" connective tissue disease. Within this "gray area" may be different subsets of fibromyalgia (see figure 1), if you want to imagine some types of fibromyalgia are more like "normal" and other types are more like "disease." There may be a hereditary susceptibility to developing this condition. Perhaps the basic cause is a change in the protein makeup of the individual, which would ultimately cause various changes in the muscles and other soft tissues, hormones and enzymes to produce fibromyalgia.

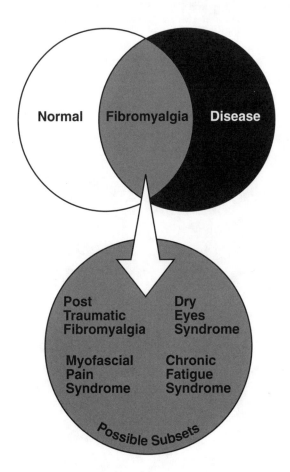

Figure 1: Fibromyalgia is a syndrome that falls in
between the high normal and low disease categories

Fibromyalgia is a unique syndrome that can be diagnosed without performing extensive and expensive tests. The main finding on physical examination is the presence of tender points that are in characteristic locations. Tender points are areas in the soft tissues, either the muscles or tendons and ligaments, which are extremely sensitive and painful when pressed and cause the individual to flinch or jump. If pressing a certain tender area causes pain, numbness or tingling to radiate to distant areas, the painful spot is called a trigger point. For example, if I press on a tender area of your back and you feel numbness radiating down your leg, that area in your back would be a trigger point. (See Figure 2)

These trigger points can cause confusion since they mimic a pinched nerve; however, the nerve is not being pinched. Rather, the sore areas of the muscles cause radiating symptoms to distant locations. Seemingly unrelated body parts are linked together neurologically because they arose from a common tissue during the body's embryonic stage. An example of this is the experience of numbness and pain in the left arm when an individual is having a heart attack. There is no problem with the left arm, per se; rather, the heart muscle is embryonically linked with the sensory nerves of the left arm, and heart muscle injury causes referred pain to the left arm. There are hundreds of potential trigger points in the body.

It is the tender point that is the key objective finding in fibromyalgia. The tender point was the main criterion used to identify fibromyalgia in a study by the American College of Rheumatology in 1990, involving 16 centers in the U.S. and Canada. According to the American College of Rheumatology criteria, fibromyalgia is diagnosed when an individual has a history of widespread pain for at least three months, and at least 11 of 18 specific tender points. This pain is considered widespread when all of the following are present: pain in both sides of the body, pain above and below the waist and pain along the spine.

9

Diagnosis of Fibromyalgia

"Learn what you are and be such."

– Pindar

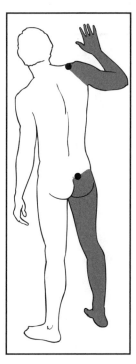

Figure 2: Tender point and radiating pain

> Fibromyalgia... can be diagnosed without performing extensive and expensive tests. The main finding on physical examination is the presence of tender points that are in characteristic locations.

The "signature" 18 tender points are located in nine areas of the body, both sides (see Figure 3). They include:

1. The occiput, or back of the head where the neck muscles connect to the skull, known as the sub-occipital muscle insertion.

2. Low cervical muscles. This is along the neck muscles in front of the fifth, sixth and seventh cervical vertebrae.

3. Trapezius muscle. This broad muscle extends from the neck to the shoulder, and the specific tender point is at the midpoint of the upper part of the muscle.

4. Supraspinatus muscle. This muscle is located in the top of the shoulder blade and should be tender on the part closer to the spine.

5. The second rib. This costochondral area is right below the collar bone.

6. Lateral epicondyle. This is located at the top of the forearm and is also called the tennis elbow area.

7. Outer gluteus maximus. This is the buttock muscle and should be tender in the upper outer portion.

8. Greater trochanter. This is part of the femur, or thigh bone, which has a knobby protrusion right below the hip joint, covered by a bursa.

9. Medial knee. This tender area is right above the inside of the knee.

Other muscle and soft tissue areas may be tender in addition to these 18 areas described in the criteria. The criteria attempt to establish strict findings for diagnosing generalized fibromyalgia in patients who have muscle pain. Although patients with fibromyalgia have particularly sensitive tender points, they also tend to be more sore all over with palpation compared to a person without fibromyalgia. A person does not need to have the required 11 tender points to be diagnosed with generalized fibromyalgia. People who

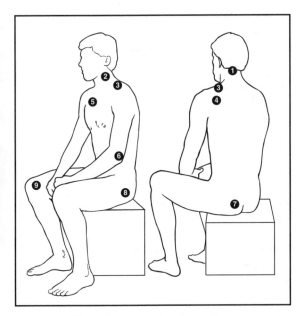

Figure 3: 18 tender points are located in nine areas of the body

have less than 11 of the required tender points may still be diagnosed as long as they have widespread pain and many of the common symptoms associated with fibromyalgia.

The fibromyalgia muscles have a peculiar consistency that feels like nylon bands when they are rubbed deeply. This band-like or ropy consistency is a characteristic feature (see Figure 4). Sometimes these

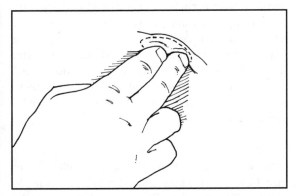

Figure 4: A fibromyalgia nodule can be palpated in the muscle

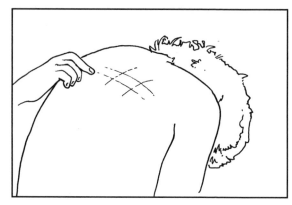

Figure 5: Dermatographia

taut bands or ropiness involve a large area, to the point where a fibromyalgia nodule, a firm lump, can be palpated in the muscles.

The skin is often hypersensitive to scratching with a finger, to the point where red marks form. This is called dermatographia, "skin writing," and it looks like someone can play tic tac toe on your back (see Figure 5). The skin hypersensitivity is attributed to a hyperactive sympathetic nervous system and it is most pronounced in the skin overlying painful muscles. Other findings of a hyperactive sympathetic nervous system are cold, sweaty hands and feet, goosebumps, and vascular rashes.

There is an art to the palpation of soft tissues, and a medical examiner who is experienced in diagnosing fibromyalgia can appreciate the tender points and changes in the muscle consistency. Although these findings may be subtle, they are definitely present and can be detected. Some examiners use devices called pain threshold meters and tissue compliance meters to gather specific objective measurements of the tender muscle areas.

Another physical exam finding is decreased joint range of motion due to painful, tense muscles. There may be diminished sensation either to light touch, pin prick, or vibration. Usually, an entire limb such as the arm or leg has sensory impairment. Muscle testing may reveal difficulty in sustaining full contractions due to muscle pain. Actual joint inflammation, specific sensory nerve loss, or true muscle weakness are not present as part of fibromyalgia, and if these abnormal physical findings are present, then they represent something other than fibromyalgia.

There seems to be a characteristic fibromyalgia posture in which the head and neck lean more forward and the shoulders are more rounded (see Figure 6). This position is our position of comfort, but over years of poor posturing, we develop more permanent structural changes in our soft tissues and bones, causing this postural deviation that can be noted on physical examination. This postural deviation is not the same as scoliosis, but as noted earlier, a separate condition of scoliosis may be seen in some people with fibromyalgia.

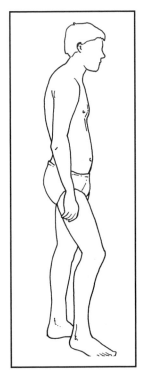

Figure 6: Fibromyalgia posture

Routine laboratory studies, x-rays, and EMGs will all be normal with this condition. No disease is found in the bones or nerves. Because routine tests are normal does not mean that fibromyalgia does not exist, or that all the tests will be normal. Sleep studies, electron microscopy studies, muscle oxygenation studies, substance P and serotonin levels, tilt table testing and other sophisticated studies have been shown to be abnormal in patients with fibromyalgia. Some of these studies are only available in a few medical centers. These tests are not considered part of the routine testing for individuals with muscle pain, even though the tests may be abnormal if the person had fibromyalgia.

Just because there are no routine lab abnormalities and "only" tender points are found, does not mean that there is no problem. As we've learned, tender points and normal routine labs are exactly what we expect to find with fibromyalgia. To an experienced examiner, tender points are the "signature" findings of fibromyalgia.

Fibromyalgia has been termed "the invisible condition" because the muscles appear normal and there are no obvious abnormalities when looking at an individual with fibromyalgia. Fibromyalgia muscles may look good on the outside, but they are definitely hurting on the inside.

10

Treatment of Fibromyalgia

Now that we know what fibromyalgia is, what can be done? The bad news is there is no known cure (yet) for this condition. The good news is that the symptoms can definitely be controlled. Fibromyalgia is not a bunch of trigger points, but rather a whole person who is having chronic muscle pain that is affecting his or her entire life. I favor an integrated, multi-level team approach in which the person with fibromyalgia is the captain of the team and is responsible for finding out what works best and integrating these positive techniques into his or her lifestyle. The rehabilitation approach focuses on one's abilities and seeks to minimize pain and maximize function. The word "habile" from "rehabilitation" means "to make able again." Even though the condition is chronic, the pain it causes can be minimized and controlled so the person can be able again.

"Care more for the individual patient than for the special features of the disease."

– Sir William Osler

There are various health professionals who treat fibromyalgia. They include family physicians, internists, physiatrists, rheumatologists, orthopedic surgeons, chiropractors, physical therapists, occupational therapists and psychologists. If certain associated conditions are major problems, other health professionals can be utilized as needed. For example, a dental referral may help if TMJ dysfunction is a problem; a gastroenterology referral may help if irritable bowel symptoms are prominent. Vocational counselors, dietitians and others can also be valuable team members in treating fibromyalgia.

The primary goal is to develop the most successful treatment possible for long-term benefit. A wide variety of treatment approaches are used involving education, medication and therapies.

Once the patient learns about and understands fibromyalgia, and is reassured that he or she is not going to die from it, then I believe over half the battle is already won. You need to learn all you can about this condition and how it affects you in your everyday life. Although you do not want to have this condition, you are stuck with it and must learn how to control it. It is your responsibility to take control of your body and your fibromyalgia.

Read all you can about fibromyalgia. Various books, brochures and newsletters are available. Your local Arthritis Foundation office has educational brochures and information about local support groups.

Excellent newsletter and reference sources are:

Fibromyalgia Network
P.O. Box 31750
Tucson, AZ 85751–1750
(800) 853-2929

The Fibromyalgia Times
P.O. Box 21990
Columbus, OH 43221–0990
(614) 457-4222

USA Fibromyalgia Association
P.O. Box 20408
Columbus, OH 43220
(614) 764-8010

Follow-up with your doctor who is treating your fibromyalgia and work together to develop the best treatment program. Your doctor and other members or your health care team will be able to make recommendations and suggestions to better control your symptoms and make sure that you are developing effective long-term strategies. Your doctor will also be able to learn from you, so share your knowledge and work together.

11

Educating Yourself about Fibromyalgia

"Pain makes man think. Thought makes man wise. Wisdom makes life endurable."

– John Patrick

There is no "magic" pill that will get rid of all fibromyalgia symptoms. Certain drugs can be very effective in reducing discomfort and improving overall feelings of well being. No one type of medication works for everyone, and no one medication causes 100% improvement. You and your doctor will have to experiment to find out what works best for you. There are various categories of drugs used in the treatment of fibromyalgia.

12
Fibromyalgia and Medications

1. **Analgesics or pain killers**. This category of medicine can include over the counter medicine such as aspirin, acetaminophen, or prescription-strength pain pills such as narcotics or central nervous system-acting drugs. These medicines do not alter the fibromyalgia condition, but they can sometimes be helpful to take the edge off pain. Narcotic medications have potential for adverse side effects, including addiction, so they should be avoided as much as possible in fibromyalgia. Over the counter pain relieving ointments, creams and gels that are rubbed into the skin can create a soothing warmth that decreases pain.

2. **Nonsteroidal anti-inflammatory drugs (NSAIDs)**. This class of medication is both anti-inflammatory (reduces inflammation) and analgesic (reduces pain). A common drug in this category is ibuprofen, which is available both over the counter and by prescription. There are numerous other medications in this group. Because fibromyalgia is not a true inflammation, these drugs are often ineffective and do not substantially reduce pain. However, these drugs can be helpful, especially if there is a flare-up that is clearly associated with excessive physical activity or if there is tendonitis or bursitis. Once the flare-up is controlled or the pain returns to the baseline level, these medications may no longer be effective and therefore should be stopped and used only as needed for flare-ups.

"The desire to take medicine is perhaps the greatest feature which distinguishes man from the animals."

– William Osler

3. **Corticosteroids**. Corticosteroids or steroids can be given by pills and by injection. Steroids are potent anti-inflammatory and analgesic medication. Whereas steroid pills have been shown to be an integral part of treatment for certain forms of inflammatory arthritis, such as rheumatoid arthritis, the long-term use of steroid pills has not been shown to be effective, nor does it have a place in the treatment of fibromyalgia. Injections of steroids for localized muscle and tendon pain have been shown to be helpful. See Chapter 13 on trigger point injections.

4. **Antidepressant medication**. There are two classes of antidepressants that are commonly used to treat fibromyalgia:

Tricyclic Antidepressants: Studies done with these drugs, particularly one called amitriptyline, have shown decreased pain in patients with fibromyalgia. In fibromyalgia, these drugs are not being used for depression, but rather to treat the fibromyalgia. Much lower doses are used to treat fibromyalgia than depression. The exact mechanism of these drugs is not known, but they have a combination of positive effects, including improved sleep, decreased pain and muscle relaxation. Because a major side effect of these medications is sedation, a low dose of the antidepressant drug is prescribed at bedtime to help improve sleep. By morning, the sedation side effect of the medicine has worn off, but the other beneficial effects of the drug continue throughout the day.

Serotonin Selective Antidepressants: As mentioned earlier, serotonin is a special type of protein, called a neurotransmitter, that is involved in the brain's regulation of pain and sleep. A deficiency or decreased effect of this neurotransmitter may play a major role in the fibromyalgia pathology, as well as causing depression. Medications that alter the serotonin concentration, by increasing either its production, its bioavailability or its effectiveness, have been used with success in the treatment of fibromyalgia.

5. **Muscle relaxants**. Drugs that cause muscle relaxation can decrease tenderness and improve pain in people with fibromyalgia. Since there appears to be increased muscle tension, especially in the sore muscles of fibromyalgia, one of the mechanisms of the muscle relaxants would be to decrease the tension and thereby decrease the pain signals.

6. **Sleep modifiers**. Since poor sleep is typical in most patients with fibromyalgia, a medication strategy includes trying to improve deep restorative sleep. Various medicines can be used that cause sedation, relaxation, or improved sleep patterns. A better quality sleep often leads to a better, less painful day.

> No one medicine will eliminate all the symptoms, but hopefully some combination of medicines will help to decrease pain, improve sleep and decrease muscle tension.

Certain medications may work well for someone else and not even touch your symptoms. No one medicine will eliminate all the symptoms, but hopefully some combination of medicines will help to decrease pain, improve sleep and decrease muscle tension. All medications have side effects, and many of them can be habit-forming or addictive if used incorrectly. You must become familiar with any potential side effects of the medication that you are taking, whether it be over-the-counter or prescription, and take only as directed by your doctor. If you ever have any questions or concerns about a particular medicine, consult with your doctor immediately.

This technique is a way of administering medicine directly into the painful tender areas of the muscles and soft tissues that are so characteristic of fibromyalgia. This technique is called trigger point injections, but more appropriately, it should be called tender and trigger point injections depending, on whether the area is a tender point or a trigger point. These injections are performed by a doctor who is experienced with fibromyalgia. The tender and trigger points causing the most problems are identified by careful palpation.

Although fibromyalgia is characterized by numerous tender points, usually six or fewer areas are causing more than 90% of the current pain. Careful palpation can localize the worst part of the tender point, which is about the size of a fingernail.

A few milliliters of medication are drawn up into a syringe. The medication may be a local anesthetic, or a local anesthetic mixed with an injectable steroid, or plain steroid alone. The medication is injected quickly into the tender point, using a small needle to minimize discomfort, and within a few moments, the patient should feel numbness and significantly reduced pain in that area. After the injections, the muscles are gently stretched to try to achieve reflex relaxation and more prolonged benefit. The injections can provide relief lasting a few days to many weeks.

The majority of people will note immediate decreased pain within a few minutes after the injection; I've only had a few individuals who reported that the injections increased their pain. There is no way of knowing how long the injections will work with any given individual, but in my experience, the average duration of benefit is about three weeks.

Trigger point injections can be especially helpful in confirming the diagnosis. For example, if your arm numbness disappears after an injection of the shoulder trigger point, even if just for a few days, then this allows your doctor to conclude that your arm symptoms are arising from the shoulder trigger point and

13

Trigger Point Injections in Fibromyalgia

"There are risks and costs to a program of action. But they are far less than the long-range risks and costs of comfortable inaction."

– John F. Kennedy

not due to a different problem. Trigger point injections are therefore helpful both from a diagnostic as well as a therapeutic standpoint. It has also been shown that trigger point injections in one area can desensitize or inactivate other tender and trigger points in the region, even though the other ones were not injected.

Trigger point injections work by desensitizing or inactivating the neurologic cycle of pain within the muscle. The local anesthetic medication is active for only a few hours but the effect on that trigger point lasts much longer, probably due to a successful long-term disruption of the reverberating cycle of pain signals. I have found local anesthetics to be most effective, but I will use steroids in combination with a local anesthetic in those regions where I feel there is an acute inflammation, such as an acute tennis elbow or bursitis. The steroid is active for days and helps resolve the acute inflammatory process.

Surprisingly, some studies have shown that just sticking a needle into the tender point without injecting any medicine, called dry needling, or injecting normal saline (physiologic salt water) can decrease pain in the tender point. What probably happens is that the needle stimulation or mechanical pressure of an injected fluid into the tender area is enough to stimulate nerve receptors to block the cycle of pain in the tender point. However, I have found injecting active medication to be far more effective than dry needling or saline shots. Fascinating research is being done using diluted botulism toxin injected into tender points. Botulism toxin causes small areas of muscle-nerve junction destruction which relaxes the affected muscle. Certain conditions such as spasmodic torticollis (wryneck), tremors and strabismus have been helped with botulism injections, and fibromyalgia tender points can also be inactivated for long periods of time with this new drug.

Remember, fibromyalgia is not a bunch of tender points. Rather, it is a whole individual whose life has been significantly affected by this syndrome.

Physical therapies are very important in the treatment of fibromyalgia. Not everyone with fibromyalgia needs physical therapy, but most of my patients have benefited. My philosophy is to develop an effective program that works best for you. Different therapies work better for different persons, and we need to determine what is best for that individual. An ideal program should be successful and easy to do; otherwise you will not do it at home.

Physical therapy consists of a wide variety of treatments including heat, cold, massage, electric stimulation, whirlpool, soft tissue mobilization exercises, stretching exercises, aerobic exercises and more. I have found that a regular stretching and flexibility program, combined with light aerobic exercises three times a week and the right mixture of heat and self massage works best for me.

Your doctor can prescribe a therapy program, which can be carried out by a trained medical professional (doctor, therapist, aide, etc.). Usually, a person is having considerable pain when he or she is first diagnosed with fibromyalgia, and the initial purpose of the therapy program is to decrease the pain using a variety of modalities. Heat is a common physical modality, and it can be given in the form of a hot pack, ultrasound, or whirlpool. Heat causes relaxation of the muscles and joints, which helps decrease pain and increase flexibility. About 20 minutes of heat application is enough to give the full benefit of heat.

Cold treatments can be just as effective in reducing pain and relaxing muscles. If a person can tolerate the first five minutes of a cold application, then he or she will be able to experience some numbness and desensitization of the skin to allow tolerance of the full 15-20 minutes of treatment. Many people have skin that is too sensitive to the cold and cannot tolerate the first five minutes. Cold can be applied by a cold pack or crushed ice in a plastic bag. The deep-muscle cooling effect of the cold modality can insulate the tissues and slow the blood flow, neurologic signals and metabolism, thereby giving a longer-acting effect than heat.

14

Physical Therapies and Fibromyalgia

"Sweat plus sacrifice equals success."

– Charles O. Finley

> Physical therapy consists of a wide variety of treatments including heat, cold, massage, electric stimulation, whirlpool, soft tissue mobilization exercises, stretching exercises, aerobic exercises and more.

Sometimes a combination of heat and cold is used for the best effect. When the person also performs an exercise program, heat modalities can be used prior to the exercise to assist in the warm-up process, and cold modalities can be used immediately after exercising to help minimize swelling and pain and assist in the warm-down and cool-down processes.

Electrical stimulation can provide relief. Various types of electrical current can be delivered to the muscles, ranging from a mini electric current that is barely felt to a stronger electrical current that causes the muscles to contract. A special type of electric stimulation is provided by a TENS (transcutaneous electrical nerve stimulator) unit. The TENS unit consists of a box about the size of a deck of cards with wires attached. A sticky pad is at the end of each wire, and these pads are stuck to painful muscle regions. An electrical current is delivered from the box through the pads, and the signal can be adjusted to provide higher intensity and pulsations. The individual perceives an electrical "buzzing" sensation that is soothing and blocks the pain sensations.

Traction is sometimes helpful in stretching and relaxing the muscles. It can be used in the neck or back. However, many patients report that traction aggravates their fibromyalgia symptoms and cannot be tolerated.

After the acute pain begins to subside, exercises can be introduced and gradually progressed as tolerated. There are a variety of exercises used in the treatment of fibromyalgia, and your doctor can determine which exercises are best for you.

Range of motion exercises help maintain joint movement, decrease stiffness and improve flexibility. These exercises are helpful in the shoulders, neck, and hips, regions where fibromyalgia muscles tend to be particularly stiff and painful.

Stretching and flexibility exercises combine range of motion with more of a gentle yet firm stretching of the muscles and joints. Two special categories include craniosacral techniques, which are helpful in patients with TMJ dysfunction and headaches, and myofascial release techniques, which emphasize stretching of the fibromyalgia tender points.

Strengthening exercises are designed to increase muscle strength. Isometric exercises (the person tightens the muscle, but does not move the joint) can be helpful if the joints are painful, because it makes the joint stronger with very little joint movement. Isokinetic or isotonic exercises (the muscles tighten using a weight or some type of resistance, and the joints move through their motion) are effective in fibromyalgia because they allow for better blood flow and oxygenation.

Aerobic exercises are those that increase the body's heart rate to a target range to achieve desired conditioning of the heart and lungs as well as the muscles. Common aerobic exercises including walking, biking, jogging, aerobics and swimming. You need to incorporate a routine aerobic exercise program into your lifestyle, and it has to be a form of exercise that is enjoyable and will be carried out. If you hate the water, a swimming program will not be for you. I hate to jog, I'm afraid of the water and I find bike riding too painful on my neck and back, so I've resorted to walking and playing basketball on a regular basis as my forms of exercise.

An excellent and safe form of exercise is water exercise, particularly aquatic or pool exercises. Exercising in the water has many benefits, even for someone who can't swim. Most of the body weight is buoyed by the water, thereby reducing the stress on the muscles and joints. The water must be kept at a comfortable temperature, usually around 85 degrees Fahrenheit, and fortunately most indoor recreational pools maintain this temperature. Cold water is our enemy! Range of motion, flexibility, strengthening and aerobic exercises can all be done in the pool and can be supervised by a trained professional until individuals feel comfortable in following

> I believe a key in the effective management of fibromyalgia is developing a successful and regular exercise program.

> Physical therapies are designed to teach you what works best and what doesn't work for you, so you can develop a successful home program.

through with their own program.

There are many proven benefits from exercise, which include decreased pain, improved flexibility, improved strength, more energy, better sleep, better weight control, improved cardiovascular fitness and improved self-esteem and feeling of well-being. I believe a key in the effective management of fibromyalgia is developing a successful and regular exercise program. Following through with a regular exercise program is always easier said than done. Your health care professionals can help guide you and supervise you in finding an exercise program that works best for you and help you integrate it into your lifestyle. The muscle pain may increase when you first start an exercise program because your muscles are not used to the stretching and activity. Your muscles have an excellent way of letting you know they don't like this increased activity by sending more pain signals!

You need to work through this initial period of exercise-induced discomfort, because once you get your muscles more fit and strong, the muscle pain will decrease and your pain baseline will lessen. The therapy program is designed to help smooth the transition into a more active exercise phase with emphasis on controlling pain.

Physical therapies are designed to teach you what works best and what doesn't work for you, so you can develop a successful home program and carry out the modalities and exercises on your own. Physical therapies are not to be continued indefinitely just because the person feels good at the time of therapy. Rather, the therapy is much more effective if it is done over a defined short term with the main emphasis placed on teaching the individual how to control this condition with a home program of modalities and exercises.

Massage has been found to be helpful in fibromyalgia. Massage consists of several techniques to help relieve muscle pain. Stroking is the gliding of palms and fingers firmly over the muscles in a slow, rhythmic movement to help decrease tension. Kneading is when the muscle is grasped between the fingers and thumb and slightly lifted and squeezed, again in a slow, rhythmic sequence. Friction massage penetrates deep into the muscles and uses slow, circular movements with the tips of the fingers or thumb.

Massage helps decrease pain by several mechanisms, including relaxing muscles, improving circulation and oxygenation, helping remove waste build-up in the muscles and making the muscles more flexible. Massage therapy can be administered by a physical therapist, massotherapist or neuromuscular therapist. Specialized massage techniques can be used successfully in treating fibromyalgia. These include strain/counterstrain (putting tissues in position of greatest comfort), soft tissue mobilization (loosening tissues and joints), trigger point therapy/shiatsu (pressure on trigger points and acupuncture points) and myofascial release (relieving spasms and tightness). The results are even better if massage therapy is combined with other forms of treatment such as moist heat and exercises.

Self massage is a simple procedure that can be learned easily to allow you to work your own muscles to achieve pain reduction and relaxation. I find self massage, particularly in my painful trapezius muscles, to be a convenient and helpful way of reducing pain, no matter where I am or what time of the day it is. A spouse or significant other can be trained how to perform therapeutic massage.

15

Massage and Fibromyalgia

"Tis the human touch in the world that counts..."

– Spencer M. Free

Osteopathic physicians and chiropractic physicians are trained to perform manipulations and adjustments. These techniques can mobilize joints, improve range of motion, relax muscles, and reduce muscle pain. All these can benefit patients with fibromyalgia.

Manipulations are forceful movements of body parts, such as the neck, to bring about a greater range of movement and relax muscles. Adjustments are the application of a sudden and precise force to a specific point in the vertebra or muscle to properly align the body. The desired outcome of properly aligned vertebrae and muscles is improved circulation and neurologic flow which reduces tension and pain.

Many chiropractors use a device called an Activator to perform adjustments. This handheld device has a spring loaded plunger mechanism which delivers focused pressure energy to a specific body part to achieve proper alignment. Many fibromyalgia patients report excellent results with this type of adjustment therapy.

As with other treatments, manipulative therapies may work well alone, but often work best when used in conjunction with other forms of treatment. Each patient with fibromyalgia needs to develop an individualized treatment regimen that works best for him or her.

16

Manipulation and Fibromyalgia

"The art of life lies in a constant readjustment to our surroundings."
– Okakura Kakuzo

Occupational therapy, often referred to as OT, can play an important role in helping patients with fibromyalgia. Occupational therapy helps one become as independent as possible with emphasis on use of the arms in a functional manner for all activities of daily living including feeding, bathing and dressing, as well as homemaking, working and leisure time activities.

In individuals with fibromyalgia, occupational therapy can concentrate on improving arm strength, coordination and ways to minimize pain and prevent the pain from interfering with functional activity. This may involve teaching the person new ways to perform various tasks including dressing, cutting potatoes, running the sweeper, using power tools, operating a computer keyboard and much more.

An occupational therapist also has training in the vocational aspect and can be a valuable team member in helping fibromyalgia patients maintain employment by successfully adapting the work setting to best suit the painful limitations caused by the fibromyalgia.

Ergonomics is a special science which involves designing work tasks to fit the capabilities of the human body. A worker with fibromyalgia can be taught to apply ergonomic techniques to minimize muscle pain or injuries.

I have coined the word "fibronomics" to describe the unique body mechanisms needed in persons with fibromyalgia. Fibronomics is defined as the art of properly manipulating our fibromyalgia bodies in the environment to enable pain-free completion of a function or activity.

17

Occupational Therapy and Fibromyalgia

"Employment is nature's physician and is essential to human happiness."

– Galen

A psychologist can be helpful in the overall management of fibromyalgia. If it is suggested that you work with a psychologist to help manage your fibromyalgia pain, that is not the same as saying the pain is "all in your head" or that you are crazy. Rather, it is the recognition that chronic painful fibromyalgia affects all of you, including your mental outlook. Physical pain can eventually cause very real psychological reactions. It is normal to become fearful, frightened, frustrated, angry, anxious and even depressed because of chronic pain. At times, these feelings can lead to decreased self-esteem and severe depression with a negative outlook.

Psychological stress not only threatens the individual's sense of stable control or balance, it also seriously threatens the interpersonal relationships with family and friends. The personal and family stress add further to the overall physical and emotional burden of fibromyalgia. The person's entire lifestyle is disrupted–striking testimony that fibromyalgia is more than a condition of painful muscles.

Psychological treatment includes a variety of programs such as psychotherapy, counseling, pain and stress management, biofeedback, relaxation, coping strategies and other techniques to improve your overall therapeutic response.

Pain management techniques teach the mind how to relax muscles, reduce pain and decrease stress and anxiety. Biofeedback is a specific technique in which individuals learn to control their body responses to achieve relaxation and pain relief. It teaches self awareness, self control and self responsibility. Various types of biofeedback and relaxation exercises can be taught, and these techniques seem to work well for over half of the patients. Not everyone can learn to relax, and that who do usually require several weeks of instruction and practice before they start to notice any benefits.

Psychotherapy or counseling can help an individual

18

Psychology and Fibromyalgia

"What you think means more than anything else in your life."

– George Matthew Adams

> Psychotherapy or counseling can help an individual overcome feelings of depression, anger and frustration.

overcome feelings of depression, anger and frustration brought upon by the fibromyalgia and associated lost abilities. Coping techniques to deal with fear of the future, job pressures and tensions, family concerns and other issues can be learned, and the individual hopefully can achieve a healthy balance.

Psychologists can help make the change from "I can't because of my fibromyalgia" to "I can in spite of my fibromyalgia."

19

Pain Is a Bad Word

Pain is a bad word. In fact it is a dirty, four-letter word. All we have to do is look in any magazine or watch TV, and we will see multiple creative ads bombarding us constantly and telling us that pain is bad and we need to take pain medication. People spend over $1 billion a year on over-the-counter drugs for pain and the cost of treatment of pain is estimated to be about $60 billion a year, which includes medical costs, lost wages and compensation.

Pain may be a warning that something is wrong, and it may invoke fear that something terrible is wrong such as a heart attack or cancer. But pain is a part of living. The average American over 45 has 2.3 painful conditions and, as you've learned, many people have fibromyalgia, too.

In prehistoric times, it was felt that pain was caused by demons entering the body through wounds and swimming around, and the treatment was to create new wounds to allow fluids with the demons to escape. During the Renaissance, the heart was perceived as the pain center. It wasn't until the 1800s that the role of the nervous system was understood as the cause of pain. We now know that pain is a complicated process of the nervous system.

Pain is a process that begins at the nerve endings of skin, muscles, bones or other tissues. Neuroreceptors can detect any noxious or painful stimulations. Chemicals called neurotransmitters create tiny electrical currents that travel up nerves into the spinal cord, where the signals are routed up specific pain tracts to the brain. It isn't until the signal reaches the brain that a phenomenon called nociperception occurs, which is when the brain detects pain, and therefore you first perceive the original signals to be painful. This whole process happens in milliseconds, so if you put your hand on a hot stove, your brain immediately perceives this to be a painful signal.

> "Pain is a part of living. It is an expected and necessary part of our interface with the environment. Pain is a privilege, a reminder of being alive."
>
> – Ernest W. Johnson, M.D.

> ...the body tries to naturally treat itself by a process called accommodation, or natural desensitization to pain, and by releasing the body's own pain medication, called endorphins.

The process from the receptors to the brain's detection of pain is constant and universal in all humans. Yet that is not the same as saying all individuals perceive pain the same way. These differences have to do with an interesting part of the brain called the limbic system, which modulates the pain responses, and specifically controls the emotional and behavioral responses to pain. Fear, anxiety and depression can modulate one's perception of how bad the pain is. One's pain threshold can be elevated or lowered based on emotional responses.

Similarly, learned responses to pain or behavioral responses can affect one's perception of pain. In America, a child learns at a very young age that a cut on the knee will result in a shower of attention, a Band-Aid, and a reward to help ease the pain. Furthermore, the Band-Aid sends a signal to everyone that elicits a typical response, "Oh, no, you got a boo-boo. How does it feel?" The child learns that pain can be rewarded with attention and other good things.

Likewise, an individual can learn to signal pain behaviors to others to indicate that the person is hurting. A facial grimace, groaning, or grabbing one's back may be signals that call others' attention to pain. If these pain behaviors or signals are used to avoid undesired chores, as an excuse not to visit in-laws, or to convince a doctor that the person is disabled from work, then the pain behaviors are being used to achieve secondary gains.

The expectation of the pain can also affect the perceived severity of pain. For example, most mothers will tell me that pregnancy ends with the worst pain they've ever experienced, yet many mothers have been pregnant many times. Why is that? Quite simply, despite the severe pain during delivery, the outcome of their pain was good, that is, a new life was born and this is a highly positive reward. On the other hand, an individual with chronic muscle pain with no end in sight may attribute their pain to be the worse imaginable because of the anticipated bad outcome or never-ending pain.

Pain is usually divided into two types, acute and chronic. Acute pain can be a brief warning signal, such as touching a hot stove with no damage done to the tissue. Or there could be tissue damage, as occurs with a muscle sprain or a bone fracture. In acute pain, healing is the expected outcome, and the pain should go away completely.

In chronic pain, either there is progression of the tissue damage, as occurs in certain types of inflammatory arthritis, or the pain signals persist even though the acute "injury" may have subsided. When pain signals are continuously sent, the body tries to naturally treat itself by a process called accommodation, or natural desensitization to pain, and by releasing the body's own pain medication, called endorphins.

> Fibromyalgia is not simply a bunch of tender points, but rather a condition that affects the whole person.

The chronic pain related to fibromyalgia consists of a complex interaction of the body's physiologic, neurologic and emotional mechanisms. The tender points may have physiologic deficiencies within the muscle and nerve endings that result in higher concentration of pain proteins (such as substance P, serotonin, and other neurotransmitters), which causes a chemical hypersensitization of the pain endings. Not only are these hypersensitive nerves more easily activated to send pain signals upward to the brain, there appears to be a loss of ability to shut off these pain signals or regulate them. Instead of the pain signal traveling up once and then stopping, it sets up a vicious cycle of repetitive pain stimulation. Consequently, the tender points are painful not only when pressed on, but also spontaneously.

Just as the tender point mechanism involves more than just the actual small area of muscle, the condition of fibromyalgia involves more than just tender points. As I've indicated earlier, fibromyalgia is not simply a bunch of tender points, but rather a condition that affects the whole person. Whereas fibromyalgia itself is not considered a disease, the associated pain and disability can cause such disruption in one's daily functional abilities that they should be regarded as a "disease."

20

Effectively Dealing with Fibromyalgia

Fibromyalgia is a syndrome that you have to live with every day. I know from personal and professional experience that this is hard, because fibromyalgia hurts. It is a part of you even though you never wanted it in the first place. You have to first learn to accept it and then to cope with it. A psychologist once affectionately likened having fibromyalgia to having a distant aunt coming to pay a visit. Her company is not necessarily welcome, she overstays her visit and her habits may be most annoying, yet she is part of your family and you try to make the best of the situation.

With fibromyalgia, the goal is not to try to completely eliminate your pain, since that rarely happens. Rather, the goal becomes: How can I learn to go on in spite of the pain and take control of this condition?

Self responsibility is necessary to fully understand and accept fibromyalgia. It is your responsibility to learn everything you can about the condition and to actively discover what works best for you in treatment. The more you know and understand about fibromyalgia, the less frightening or unbearable it becomes.

Being self responsible means accepting that this condition is part of you and that it is a permanent condition. Even if we do not know the exact cause, we know a lot about this syndrome. We also know that there is no cure. There are various factors that precipitate fibromyalgia, but stress is not a cause, so we can't blame stress. It is impossible to eliminate stress in one's life. Life, by definition, is stressful! You can learn how to modify or minimize stress to help better control your fibromyalgia.

Part of being self responsible is increasing others' awareness, particularly that of family, friends and employers. Since you look normal, others can't "see" your invisible condition and hidden pain. Fibromyalgia is not a topic that everyone under-

> "To strive with difficulties and to conquer them is the highest human felicity."
>
> – Samuel Johnson

> It is possible to develop a positive strategy in effectively dealing with fibromyalgia.

stands or one that invokes immediate empathy and compassion such as cancer pain or heart attack pain. We need to help others understand what you are going through with fibromyalgia to allow empathy and compassion, but not sympathy.

Another key part of self responsibility is following through with your treatment program. It takes a lot of work on your part to deal with fibromyalgia, and you need to work hard at it every day. You are the captain of a team of consultants who will help you deal with your fibromyalgia, and it is up to you to responsibly carry out the recommendations.

Finally, part of the self responsibility of fibromyalgia is having realistic expectations. Your condition causes very real functional limitations and pain. If you expect that the treatments directed at fibromyalgia will leave you completely pain-free, your expectations are unrealistic. If you expect that your condition will go away over time once you find the right pill or right magical bullet, you are having unrealistic expectations. You should have hope that someday a cure will be discovered, but you have to balance this hope with a realistic approach to your current everyday life, including the adjustments that need to be made in order to deal with fibromyalgia.

It is possible to develop a positive strategy in effectively dealing with fibromyalgia. You've got it, so you might as well accept it and do something about it. We medical professionals are here to help you, but you have to live your own life. Help is available, but you must take a positive attitude and be responsible for trying to improve your situation.

There is no one magical treatment for fibromyalgia; you need to determine what works best for you. It will usually be a combination of modalities, stretching exercises and aerobic exercises. Some people like heat, so they use heating pads, hot showers, hot packs or a heating lamp at home. Various muscle creams can be applied to provide chemical heat. Others prefer cold, so home ice packs or ice massages can be helpful. Almost everyone benefits from massage, either self massage or from a significant other, and stretching exercises can be easily taught. Your doctor can help you set up an effective and inexpensive home program.

You need to increase your overall level of fitness. An aerobic exercise program such as walking, swimming (preferably in a heated pool), aerobic dancing and recreational sports is probably the single most effective treatment for fibromyalgia. It benefits you both physically and psychologically, and you owe it to yourself to take time out and take care of yourself. Most people with fibromyalgia allow their muscles to become chronically unfit through disuse. General strengthening and aerobic exercises to start can usually ease the fibromyalgia pain symptoms, but expect your muscles to hurt at first as you work through the deconditioning. A temporary increase in pain is common and does not mean you are getting worse.

Each person, through trial and error, must determine his or her own "fine line" between how much exercise is helpful and how much is causing a flare-up of symptoms. There is no question that a regular exercise program is difficult to incorporate into one's lifestyle, but it is absolutely necessary in the long term treatment of fibromyalgia. In the long term, exercises will decrease, not increase, pain. Even if you hurt, you should still do exercises, because they won't harm you or make your condition worse. On the other hand, if you don't do your exercises regularly, you will be far more likely to have a higher level of pain and more flare-ups.

21

Developing an Effective Home Program

"Do what you can, with what you have, where you are."

– Theodore Roosevelt

> General strengthening and aerobic exercises to start can usually ease the fibromyalgia pain symptoms, but expect your muscles to hurt at first.

Non-traditional, or alternative therapies, may be part of one's program. Numerous alternative therapies have been used successfully in treating fibromyalgia and include chiropractic treatment, acupuncture, biomagnetic therapy, nutritional therapy, meditation, and more. I feel a blend of all treatments, traditional and alternative, works best, and each person needs to find his or her unique combination.

I learned a long time ago that not doing exercises is much worse than doing exercises when I have more pain. I need to continue with regular exercises to keep my muscles at a regular level of conditioning. If I have increased pain and do not do my exercises, I would hurt just as much as if I did do my exercises, so I feel I might as well continue to do my exercises. I know that if my muscles drop to a lower level of fitness due to inactivity, I will have far more flare-ups and pain, making it even more difficult to motivate myself to work through this pain and resume a regular exercise program. In the end, stronger painful muscles are much better than weaker painful muscles.

Every individual with fibromyalgia should be able to achieve a realistic baseline. Baseline is not the same as no pain: rather it is somewhere between no pain and the worst pain, with the primary goal of achieving a baseline as close to no pain as possible (See Figure 7). Baseline level will be different for everyone, but each person can eventually learn what his or her baseline state will be.

The baseline state is not a perfect state. That is, there are fluctuations above and below the baseline; some days you feel better and other days you feel worse. You try to have more good days than bad days, but recognize that part of fibromyalgia is having bad days or flare-ups.

Usually by the time an individual sees a doctor because of pain and receives the diagnosis of fibromyalgia, he or she has a higher level of pain. The chances are good that the program your doctor outlines for you, which can include a combination of medicine, therapy, soft tissue mobility and other techniques, will reduce your pain to a lower level. Once your pain is reduced to a lower level, you need to practice your learned techniques and carry out your home program to keep your symptoms under control.

You should strive to reduce the stress factors that may exacerbate your symptoms. Is your office desk

22

Baselines and Flare-ups

"Life is made up of sobs, sniffles, and smiles, with sniffles predominating."

– O. Henry

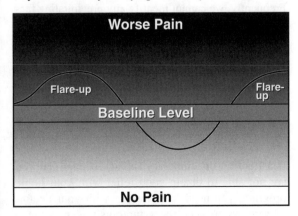

Figure 7: Baseline of pain

> We can even learn to identify subtle, yet significant, factors causing our flare-ups.

right under the air conditioner draft? Is your chair causing uncomfortable low back posturing? Are you sleeping in an uncomfortable position? Are there emotional stresses that can be reduced? Are legal battles over your fibromyalgia causing a great deal of stress? Ask yourself questions about every single thing you do during the day, trying to focus on how each activity may be contributing to your fibromyalgia symptoms. Then do something about them if you can, or ask questions if you're not sure if you can.

No matter how successful you are in developing an effective home program, no matter how stable or how prolonged your current baseline state may be, you will experience a flare-up. Unfortunately, fibromyalgia flare-ups cannot be avoided. Flare-ups can occur a few times a year or monthly, and part of dealing with flare-ups is to identify what is causing them in the first place.

You've already learned about various factors that can cause flare-ups. Many times, we can identify a certain strenuous activity that we did to cause the flare-up. As we develop more sophisticated knowledge about fibromyalgia, we can even learn to identify subtle, yet significant, factors causing our flare-ups, such as driving with the car air conditioner draft hitting our neck.

Frequently, we cannot identify any precipitating factor triggering our flare-up. This is most frustrating, especially if we've taken all the necessary steps to control our pain and prevent flare-ups. Spontaneous or idiopathic flare-ups (with no aggravation) are common and are part of fibromyalgia. If we make our best effort to control the things we can control and accept that there are uncontrollable elements, it will help us better overcome a spontaneous flare-up.

If a flare-up or temporary setback occurs and you are not able to obtain good relief with your home program, you need to follow up with your doctor. Always try to keep the symptoms under as much control as possible by yourself, but if the symptoms get out of control, you may require medications, trigger point injections, therapy or some other form of supervised treatment to help your pain return to baseline level, or to the point where you can control it again on your own.

> If we make our best effort to control the things we can control and accept that there are uncontrollable elements, it will help us better overcome a spontaneous flare-up.

It is hard to imagine that pain could ever be considered "good." Our culture is preoccupied with pain and attempts to eliminate pain. If we can't eliminate pain with medication, then we try to fool pain into being less painful by surrounding ourselves with pleasurable company, watching TV or listening to music to distract our minds. Those of us with fibromyalgia are so used to having pain that it is actually possible to categorize pain into good pain and bad pain.

The key issue is control. If we have control over our own pain level, then we are better able to deal with the consequences of the expected pain. If we know that planting a vegetable garden one spring weekend will aggravate our pain the next day, then we are in control of that pain to the extent that we can choose to plant the garden or choose not to plant the garden.

On the other hand, unexpected, unrelenting and unexplainable pain is considered bad pain. If we wake up with unexplained extreme pain or have a spontaneous flare-up, part of the "badness" of the pain is the fact that we have no control over this pain, or worse yet, we did everything we could to prevent the pain from getting worse, and it still happened.

Good pain is considered an acceptable consequence of doing something we wanted to do. We may remember that before our fibromyalgia (a long time ago!), when we would get muscle soreness following a particularly good workout. This pain was not considered too unpleasant because it reflected an activity that we enjoyed doing, and the sore muscles were actually a "reward" for our efforts.

Since we've been diagnosed with fibromyalgia, the post-exercise pains are more severe and last longer. We may feel that fibromyalgia prevents us from doing any enjoyable activities, but that is not true.

Many times, we may be in a position to choose to do

23

Good Vs. Bad Pain

"Pain is inevitable. Suffering is optional."

– Unknown

> The key issue is control. If we have control over our own pain level, then we are better able to deal with the consequences of the expected pain.

an activity even though we recognize that it may cause a flare-up. This is the concept of good pain. If you like to bowl and feel that the enjoyment from bowling outweighs the increased muscle pain that the bowling causes, then you may choose to bowl and accept the consequences. It is better to make responsible choices despite having fibromyalgia than to use fibromyalgia as an excuse to evade responsibility. You can eventually learn to appreciate the increased pain from your choices as an indication of your ability to still live your own life.

Many conditions can cause muscle pain, and you need to have a proper medical evaluation by a doctor to determine your diagnosis. If your doctor is familiar with fibromyalgia, he or she will be able to make the diagnosis. There may be laboratory studies or x-rays ordered to exclude other conditions, but fibromyalgia is a diagnosis that can be made based on the history and clinical exam.

If you wish a second opinion from another doctor, your first doctor may recommend a consulting physician. Usually a second opinion will confirm the diagnosis of fibromyalgia. Do not "doctor shop" for magic cures or miraculous surgery; there are none. Your best bet would be to work with one doctor who is completely familiar with fibromyalgia.

Treatment of fibromyalgia is not limited to only one type of doctor specialist. Many types of doctors are well trained in diagnosing and treating fibromyalgia. Specific types of doctors who see a lot of patients with fibromyalgia include physiatrists (physical medicine and rehabilitation; my specialty), rheumatologists, orthopedists, chiropractors, and primary care specialists.

In order for your doctor to help you, you need to explain your symptoms as honestly as you can. Write down notes prior to seeing your doctor. Try to be very specific about where you have pain, what part of your body it affects and what makes your pain better or worse. Tell your doctor what tests and treatments you have already had and what it is you hope to accomplish by working with him or her. Your doctor will ask you to share important personal and social aspects of your life, and how they may be part of your whole pain problem.

Ask questions and take notes. Make sure you ask for an explanation, particularly if you don't fully understand a certain subject. There is so much to learn about fibromyalgia that you could not possibly learn everything on the first visit, so you will have

24

Working with Your Doctor

"It seems sometimes as if one were powerless to do any more from within to overcome troubles, and that help must come from without."

– Arthur Christopher Benson

> Needless to say, it is important to follow through with your doctor's recommended treatment program.

opportunities during follow-up visits to get further clarifications and learn further information.

Needless to say, it is important to follow through with your doctor's recommended treatment program after the two of you have reviewed your condition and the treatment program. If you are taking medications, observe for any side effects. If you notice any unusual side effects related to your medications, stop taking the medicine and call your doctor. Never experiment with medication on your own without first discussing it with, and getting approval from, your doctor.

Do not change or stop your treatment program simply because the first few treatments or doses are not helping. Fibromyalgia is not a condition that developed overnight, so the treatment may take a while to work. You have to be patient with the treatment program, and you may need to make several adjustments along the way until your best program is achieved. Changes in your program need to be coordinated between you and your doctor, and not made indiscriminately on your own.

By taking a responsible and active role in your own medical care, you can help your doctor help you. An honest doctor-patient relationship is a successful one.

A support group can be a valuable form of treatment in fibromyalgia. Having the opportunity to share your experiences with someone else who knows exactly how you feel can be a powerful form of therapy. We in the medical profession recognize that all of our modern medicines and treatments may not be enough; an entirely different dimension of effective therapy can be provided by a support group.

A support group consists of individuals who share a common problem, fibromyalgia, and who are interested in meeting on a regular basis to share information and experiences. A successful support group usually will consist of between 10 and 20 members. Of that group there are individuals with newly-diagnosed fibromyalgia who are in the early stages of accepting and coping with their condition and in need of guidance and support from more experienced members. Others in the group have more experience in dealing with fibromyalgia and can relate to the newer members, yet still learn from the more regular members. Other regular members have reached a balance in successfully dealing with fibromyalgia, and they are interested in sharing their experiences to help others achieve a similar level.

Several years ago, many of my patients with fibromyalgia expressed an interest in forming a fibromyalgia support group. With the help of a psychologist, we organized a group that has been meeting on a monthly basis ever since. My interests are both personal and professional, and my involvement with the support group includes not only being an active participant, but also being a professional advisor. The psychologist serves as a group facilitator and has been superb. Our group has been fortunate to have wonderful people who are committed to making this group a successful one.

Our support group meets on a monthly basis for two hours; the first hour is usually devoted to education, and the second hour is devoted to support. Educational sessions have included inviting guest speakers on physical therapy, massotherapy, neuro-

25

The Value of a Fibromyalgia Support Group

"Life can only be understood backwards; but it must be lived forwards."

– Soren Kierkegaard

> A support group consists of individuals who share a common problem, fibromyalgia, and who are interested in meeting on a regular basis to share information and experiences.

muscular therapy, chiropractic treatment, new types of treatments and much more.

By far the most rewarding and successful component of this support group is the actual support component. Each individual states his or her name and shares information about life with fibromyalgia. Individuals who have had particularly difficult times in the past month may discuss their difficulties, and the rest of the group will try to provide helpful insight and share experiences to help these individuals more effectively cope with their situation. Likewise, if an individual is doing particularly well, the group wants to hear that as well so they can feel glad for the individual.

Frequently heard comments from support group participants include, "I never realized that there were others who knew exactly how I feel," or "I thought I had it bad, now I realize others have it worse than me." Those who participate in a support group are most appreciative of the opportunity. The ones who keep coming back are the ones who are benefiting from the group.

Tears of happiness and sadness are common in a support group and a successful support group makes everyone feel welcome and willing to share innermost feelings and fears.

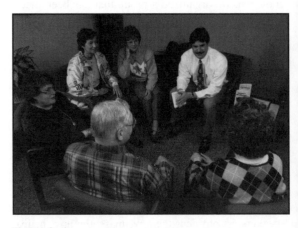

Figure 8: A support group meeting

Not everyone is a candidate for a support group. Many people with fibromyalgia are not comfortable or are not interested in sharing their experiences in a group setting. Many individuals find a support group very helpful at first, and then, once they develop good coping strategies, no longer feel a support group is needed. I invite everyone with fibromyalgia to attend a support group to see if they may benefit from this type of approach.

Having the opportunity to share your experiences with someone else who knows exactly how you feel can be a powerful form of therapy.

Once you've learned about fibromyalgia, you should evaluate every single thing you do in your day while focusing on how everything you do may affect your fibromyalgia. At first, you need to force yourself to consciously think of what you do, how you sleep, what you eat, how you hold the phone and so on. Once you've consciously identified potential problems, they can be consciously corrected. If consciously repeated enough times, these altered behaviors that better suit your fibromyalgia will eventually become part of your subconscious, and you will automatically carry out these behaviors without having to think about them.

Fibromyalgia and sleep

Since fibromyalgia interferes with our sleep, especially the deep sleep stage, we need to devise strategies to ensure the best and most restful sleep. It is during sleep that our body repairs itself, makes vital proteins and replenishes our energy supply.

It is important to develop a routine sleep schedule where you go to bed and get up at the same times. Studies have shown that if you want extra sleep, it is better to go to bed earlier rather than sleeping in later. What you do prior to going to bed is also part of the sleep routine. Do something relaxing before going to bed like listening to music, reading a book or watching a TV program. Practice some of the relaxation techniques you have learned. Avoid caffeine in the evening.

I have found the most comfortable bed for fibromyalgia is one that has a good firm mattress with a soft mattress pad. This type of mattress provides good support to the spine, but also provides some cushion effect on the skin. An eggcrate mattress can be very comfortable. Many people report waterbeds to be more difficult since they are hard to get in and out of, and they do not seem to support the spine as well. An electric mattress pad or electric blanket, used properly, can produce soothing warmth while sleeping especially since we fibromyalgics are always cold. Most of us require a

26

Adjusting Your Lifestyle

"There is only one success; to be able to spend your life in your own way."

– Christopher Morley

> Once you've consciously identified potential problems, they can be consciously corrected.

sheet, even on the hottest nights, because we always get cold. I personally can't sleep unless I'm wearing socks because I will be bothered by cold feet.

The best sleeping position is the fetal position. This is a side-lying position in which your knees are bent up and your neck is bent down. A pillow should be placed between the knees to properly align the hips and pelvis, to reduce stress and increase comfort. A head pillow should be used that is not so fluffy as to push your neck upward in an unnatural position, yet not so flimsy that your head sinks down too much, but just right so that your head is in a neutral position or centered between your shoulders when you are lying on your side.

It can take a few weeks to learn to sleep in this new position, but once you become accustomed to this change, you will likely find it most beneficial and least painful. Your body will adapt to the best sleeping position as there is no one right way for everyone. I used to sleep on my stomach. Once I realized that instead of resting and relaxing my back muscles through the night, I was actually aggravating them more, thereby increasing pain, I made the switch to the side lying fetal position. It took me a week to switch, but now I am used to this position and can no longer lie on my stomach to sleep. Invariably, my pillows end up on the floor during the night, but at least I'm maintaining a comfortable and neutral position in my joints and spine.

There are multiple medications that are used to treat the sleep disorder of fibromyalgia. Some of these medications can be habit-forming, but if the sleep medicines are used as prescribed and used judiciously, very rarely is there any problem with habituation or side effects. Since fibromyalgia is a chronic condition, and the associated sleep disorder is likewise chronic, an individual is justified in taking a nightly medicine to correct the sleep disorder as long as the beneficial effects far outweigh the potential risks.

I advise my patients to use sleeping medicines only

as needed, such as during a flare-up or if there has been a particular period of poor sleep, but to try to avoid using sleeping medicines on a regular basis. The less often one uses a sleeping medicine, the more the body will respond to this medicine when you do take it, and the less chance there is of developing a tolerance to the medicine. Some people do best with a medicine nightly, and as long as the medicine is being used responsibly, I do not have any problem with this approach.

Fibromyalgia and Diet

Fibromyalgia has not been found to be caused by a vitamin deficiency, an excessive intake of certain foods, or allergies to food products. Some of my patients have identified a particular food substance such as sugar or citrus fruits that makes their fibromyalgia worse, and they tell me that discontinuing this particular food product helped to significantly lessen their symptoms.

> No food or diet will cure your fibromyalgia, but eating properly can make you healthier and feel more energetic and help in your everyday battle against fibromyalgia.

I am asked frequently whether there is any special diet for fibromyalgia. I recommend that you approach your diet by using good common sense. Keeping your weight under control will also help you feel healthier and more energetic. Less weight on the muscles also means less muscle pain. With fibromyalgia, a sound nutritional strategy includes consuming a diet low in fat and high in natural fiber. Adequate proteins and natural (not refined) carbohydrates are important, as well as watching caffeine, alcohol, and NutraSweet™.

Studies have shown that certain vitamins and minerals such as magnesium and malic acid can help decrease pain and improve energy in patients with fibromyalgia. I usually recommend nutritional supplements that include various components such as magnesium, malic acid, manganese, vitamin B1 and vitamin B6.

No food or diet will cure your fibromyalgia, but eating properly can make you healthier and feel more energetic and help in your everyday battle against fibromyalgia.

Fibromyalgia and Smoking

Smoking is bad for many reasons, but there are two reasons in particular why smoking aggravates fibromyalgia. First, the nicotine in the smoke causes constriction of the blood vessels and decreases blood flow and oxygen and nutrients to the muscles, thereby increasing pain and muscle tension. Secondly, the carbon monoxide in the smoke entering the blood stream binds to the hemoglobin molecules in the blood, and blocks oxygen from binding to the hemoglobin, thereby decreasing oxygen availability to the muscles and increasing pain. Numerous patients have told me they had impressive decrease in their pain when they stopped smoking. Your doctor may prescribe a nicotine patch for you to help you stop smoking.

Fibromyalgia and your new car

One of the most common causes of posttraumatic fibromyalgia is a whiplash injury in which the head violently jerks back and forward, usually following "minor" rear end collisions. Many times, the car head rest is ineffective in preventing or minimizing a whiplash-type injury because it is not in the right position, or it's not designed well. When looking for a new car, pay special attention to the head rest and make sure that when you are seated, the head rest can be adjusted to the middle of your head and prevent extreme backward movement of the head in the event of a rear collision. Cars with adjustable seats and backs are preferred, to enable your back to be in a comfortable position while driving and to allow changes in position that your body may require. Some cars are equipped with lumbar supports. If low back pain is a particular problem, lumbar cushions or specially designed inserts can be used.

Fibromyalgia and the home

Housework enemy number one in people with

> Numerous patients have told me they had impressive decrease in their pain when they stopped smoking.

fibromyalgia is running the sweeper. Whoever designed sweepers did not have people with fibromyalgia in mind. The reaching and pulling puts considerable stress on our painful neck and shoulder muscles, and often this activity cannot be performed at all. There are exceptionally lightweight sweeper models on the market now, and one can learn to use a sweeper while keeping the elbows to the side and transmitting the weight and force through the body, and not through the arm itself when running the sweeper.

> Try to use gravity whenever possible when doing home-making activities, instead of fighting against gravity.

Try to use gravity whenever possible when doing homemaking activities, instead of fighting against gravity. Arrange the items in your kitchen so you don't have to reach or lift overhead frequently, especially to get everyday items. Try to "neutralize" your work station to avoid excessive reaching, lifting or bending. Your furniture should be comfortable yet provide enough support to your body. Make sure that your head isn't turned in an awkward position when watching TV, talking on the phone or reading. Be especially cautious of your posture when performing enjoyable hobbies since you will be less likely to be monitoring your posture and early pain signals that may indicate that you are not in the optimum position.

Fibromyalgia and the job

Occupations that are at higher risk for causing fibromyalgia include assembly line jobs that require repetitive arm motions and clerical jobs that involve typing and computer work. The primary mechanism for this form of posttraumatic fibromyalgia is a cumulative "wear and tear" or strain-type injury to the muscles, which eventually develop fibromyalgia. An awareness of proper body posture at work and an understanding of ergonomics (using the body in its most effective and efficient manner to perform job tasks) can help reduce the job-related aggravation of your condition. Your doctor and therapists can help you develop job strategies to minimize the chance of a flare-up and help you successfully remain on the job.

Sometimes fibromyalgia can become so severe due to the job activities that the person is no longer able to continue working at that particular job because of pain. Your doctor can work with you to help you determine what your limitations are and try to help you find gainful employment at a different type of job within these limitations.

Fibromyalgia and the new mother or father

Becoming a new mother or father is certainly a joyful occasion, but it can also cause painful flare-ups of fibromyalgia. New mothers are more vulnerable to back muscle strain during pregnancy due to the increased pressure on the low back as the fetus grows bigger and heavier. The physiologic weight gain during pregnancy can also be a nuisance to fibromyalgia, and particularly for mothers who nurse, the extra breast weight can cause increased neck and shoulder pain as well as increasing the force on the low back.

The new mother is particularly challenged by the infant. This loveable, irresistible little person who weighs less than 10 pounds always manages to locate himself or herself in strategic positions that are most challenging to the new mother's ability to maintain proper spine posture. Picking the baby up from a crib or off the floor, carrying the infant, or twisting and reaching to put the infant in the car are hazards to a new mother's back and increase the risk of a flare-up of the overall fibromyalgia.

Paying special attention to proper posture, making sure that regular exercises are resumed, and allowing time for relaxation can help the new mother prevent flare-ups.

New fathers with fibromyalgia need to pay special attention since they too are vulnerable to flare-ups from challenging postures.

Posttraumatic fibromyalgia is a special subtype of fibromyalgia. Because it is so common, an entire chapter has been devoted to this special category. As the name indicates, it is the type of fibromyalgia that is caused by trauma. Trauma can be macroscopic, as in sudden forceful injury or strain to the muscle, or microscopic, such as the cumulative, repetitive, low-grade trauma over time.

The trauma may be from an obvious injury, such as occurs in a motor vehicle accident in which the body gets jerked around, resulting in muscle and soft tissue injuries. Whiplash is an example of a neck and shoulder soft tissue injury that frequently occurs during a rear-end collision. The trauma may also be more subtle, as could occur with someone who works on an assembly line all day and does a lot of reaching and pushing. These activities put minor yet cumulative strains on the neck and shoulder muscles that, over time, can lead to changes within the muscle that are seen with fibromyalgia.

The pain and tender points are the same in posttraumatic fibromyalgia as in generalized fibromyalgia syndrome. The big difference, however, is that individuals with posttraumatic fibromyalgia have pain and tender points localized to the region of their injury rather than in a generalized distribution. Consequently, the criteria for generalized fibromyalgia syndrome as set by the American College of Rheumatologists (11 of 18 tender points) may not be met. This does not mean the person does not have fibromyalgia; it simply means that the person has a more localized form of fibromyalgia caused by trauma. Some people also use the term "post-traumatic regional myofascial pain syndrome" which I believe is interchangeable with "posttraumatic regional fibromyalgia."

Why do some people get posttraumatic fibromyalgia, whereas others exposed to the same trauma do not? We do not know the exact reason, but I believe that genetic susceptibility or vulnerability plays a key role.

27

Post-traumatic Fibromyalgia

"One cannot get through life without pain... What we can do is choose how to use the pain life presents to us."

– Bernie S. Siegel, M.D.

> Once the soft tissues are traumatized...the previous pain-free "balance" is forever disrupted.

Since I believe that genetic predisposition is an important factor in determining who is going to get generalized fibromyalgia, the same logic would apply to those who are more susceptible to getting posttraumatic fibromyalgia. The vulnerable person may not have any symptoms whatsoever of fibromyalgia even though the muscles are susceptible to this condition.

These susceptible muscles and soft tissues are functioning adequately and are not painful. Once the soft tissues are traumatized, the altered pain responses are triggered, and the previous pain-free "balance" is forever disrupted, resulting in a permanently altered "balance" that is now painful. The muscles were pushed over the edge, so to speak.

A way to understand this mechanism is to imagine the changes in the muscles as a physiologic scar. Some people form abnormally prominent thick scars after they cut their skin instead of the normal thin, flat, barely perceptible scar. These people are genetically more susceptible to forming these large scars, which are called keloid scars. Using the same analogy, an individual with fibromyalgia or fibromyalgia tendencies will form an abnormal physiologic scar in the muscles after an injury. The muscles heal over time following the injury, but the neurophysiologic mechanism is not quite the same and acts differently, as if it is scarred. If the pain symptoms last longer than four to six months after an injury, they are likely to be permanent.

We have no way of predicting who is vulnerable. We also have no way of knowing who would have gone on to develop the generalized fibromyalgia over time had their course not been "interrupted" by the trauma. Some people may have gone onto develop symptoms of generalized fibromyalgia had they never had the trauma, whereas others may have never had any chronic muscle soreness had it not been for the trauma. Still others have pre-existing fibromyalgia and then are involved in an accident in which certain areas are injured, and subsequently these areas become more painful than would have occurred with the "natural" fibromyalgia course.

My fibromyalgia developed gradually over time, first involving my neck and shoulder, then my low back. No specific precipitating trauma occurred in my situation. However, my right shoulder was the first area to become painful and has been the most severe region of pain over the years. As I look back, I wonder if my job as a paper boy in my early teens may have been related. I had 100 customers on my route, and I remember that the paper bag was quite heavy stuffed with these papers, and that I always slung the strap over my right shoulder.

> We...have no way of knowing who would have gone on to develop the generalized fibromyalgia over time had their course not been "interrupted" by the trauma.

It may have been the cumulative localized trauma of the heavy paper bag pressing down on my right shoulder muscles that caused muscle changes and led to a particularly painful fibromyalgia area. Over the years, I've noticed that new areas of chronic pain were caused by a specific injury. For example, I injured my low back during basketball and developed chronically painful lumbosacral pain.

Even though my fibromyalgia symptoms did not fully express themselves until my mid-twenties, I have no doubt that if I had been involved in a motor vehicle accident when I was 18 and suffered a whiplash and other soft tissue injuries, I would have developed post traumatic fibromyalgia at that time.

Clearly, the history of how the pain problems began differs in the patient presenting to my office with generalized fibromyalgia compared to the patient with posttraumatic fibromyalgia. In generalized fibromyalgia, patients will usually describe a gradual progression of pain, usually in a few regions at first and then becoming more generalized. By the time they present for medical evaluation, they have the full-blown generalized fibromyalgia with the associated conditions such as headaches, irritable bowel syndrome, etc.

On the other hand, patients with posttraumatic fibromyalgia will usually state that they had no problems with pain until their injury, and since the injury, they have been bothered by chronic pain in the injured soft tissues. The associated conditions are not typically seen in posttraumatic fibromyalgia. Those with posttraumatic fibromyalgia have a condition that is just as chronic and permanent as the generalized fibromyalgia, and their condition also requires medical treatments and a dedicated home program. These individuals have periodic exacerbations and flare-ups also.

I have also observed that persons with posttraumatic fibromyalgia develop more generalization of their pain over time. For example, a person who had a whiplash injury and was bothered by chronic neck and shoulder pain due to posttraumatic fibromyalgia may start developing low back pain or pain in areas that were never injured by the original accident. Similarly, a factory worker who lifted a box and experienced a low back strain may, over time, start experiencing neck and shoulder pain.

If these particular individuals are evaluated by a doctor, not only will generalized painful tender points be found, but these persons will be meeting the criteria for the diagnosis of fibromyalgia as set forth by the American College of Rheumatology. In addition to the multiple painful tender points, I've had numerous patients develop irritable bowel syndrome, migraine headaches, and other associated conditions months and years after the trauma.

How can a localized posttraumatic fibromyalgia evolve into a generalized systemic fibromyalgia? There are multiple reasons this can happen. First, the patient may later experience different injuries to these different areas, causing new pain. Secondly, the person may have been destined to develop fibromyalgia anyway, and with the natural course of time, more areas are undergoing the changes that cause them to be chronically painful. Thirdly, the person may be creating unusual mechanical stresses on other muscles as these muscles are used more to compensate for or overcome the effects of the painful muscle. This mechanical microtrauma effect can involve muscles that are seemingly far away from the originally injured muscles. Lastly, there may be a neurologic mechanism occurring at the brain or spinal cord level that causes distant areas to become more painful.

From a functional standpoint, it is difficult to separate the neck from the low back, since they are both parts of the spine and the spine acts in an integrated functional manner. If an injury occurs to the lower back, it follows that the whole functional spine reacts to this injury. One of the ways it can react is to start assimilating all of these pain signals that are chronically a rising from the low back into a new nerve pattern for the brain and spinal cord.

This new nerve pattern may now "see" the entire functional unit of neck and low back, not just the low back, as "affected." What follows is a gradual yet irreversible change in the muscle and nerve physiology that we ultimately recognize as a more generalized fibromyalgia. A similar mechanism may be that the individual with fibromyalgia has a predisposed state, and once the central nervous system begins seeing altered signals from one region, this triggers a more generalized reaction.

Probably all of these factors in combination are responsible for this phenomenon. The majority of people with posttraumatic fibromyalgia do not go on to develop a generalized fibromyalgia. Localized posttraumatic fibromyalgia is essentially the same as posttraumatic myofascial pain syndrome. Whatever the name, and whatever the etiology, the treatment goals are the same: to reduce pain, improve function, and develop effective ways to prevent or minimize flare-ups.

> The treatment goals are the same: to reduce pain, improve function, and develop effective ways to prevent or minimize flare-ups.

Fibromyalgia is recognized by the courts, Worker's Compensation, and Social Security as a bonafide medical condition. Depending on how a given individual is affected by fibromyalgia and the severity of the syndrome, this recognition does not necessarily mean reimbursement. In the courts, there have been financial settlements varying from very little to large amounts. The difference is often not related to the severity of the fibromyalgia, but how convincingly one side or the other presents its case to the judge or jury regarding pain and suffering from posttraumatic fibromyalgia.

Various percentages of disability have been awarded in the Social Security and Worker's Compensation systems, with wide variations occurring among regions, states and various evaluating individuals. If fibromyalgia was activated or caused by trauma, then often the legal system will get involved, either through the courts or the Worker's Compensation system.

Individuals with posttraumatic fibromyalgia often accumulate extensive medical bills and see various doctors in order to get their condition diagnosed and treated. If the medical costs are not reimbursed by the insurance company, then a personal injury lawsuit may be filed and could ultimately end up in an actual court case. The usual issue is how much should someone be financially responsible for causing someone else's posttraumatic fibromyalgia? Both liability and compensation issues are argued.

The injured individual will be represented by a plaintiff's attorney, who should be experienced in chronic soft tissue problems, particularly posttraumatic fibromyalgia. The role of the plaintiff's attorney is to convince the judge or jury that the injured client has a chronic painful condition that cannot be cured and will always require some form of medical treatment.

The attorney will also argue that this painful condition was directly caused by the automobile accident

28

Legal Aspects and Fibromyalgia

"The law is not an end to itself, nor does it provide ends. It is preeminently a means to serve what we think is right."

– Justice William J. Brennan, Jr.

> The defense's medical witness may indicate that the fibromyalgia was a preexisting condition...and that the single trauma cannot be blamed for the individual's current problems.

and has left the individual with permanent functional impairment and a disrupted lifestyle.

The defense attorney represents the insurance company or the individual who caused the motor vehicle accident. The defense attorney usually presents a case to minimize the impact of fibromyalgia. Strategies that I've seen have included questioning the existence of fibromyalgia and whether trauma can cause it, downplaying the severity of fibromyalgia and focusing on the lack of abnormalities on the x-rays, laboratory studies and electrical studies. The injured individual, the defense may point out, has not had a serious injury, and soft tissue injuries cause no more pain than the usual pains in ordinary life.

Both attorneys will call in their expert medical witnesses, who usually testify to opposite opinions. The plaintiff's expert doctor will testify to the existence of fibromyalgia, how it causes severe muscle pain even though it can't be seen, and that it can be reproduced by objective findings, including tender points, muscle spasms, muscle ropiness, skin color changes, decreased joint motion and sensory loss.

The defense's expert doctor may indicate that there is no objective evidence of disease, and point out that fibromyalgia is a controversial condition, that there is no basis for the individual's chronic pain. The defense's medical witness may indicate that the fibromyalgia was a preexisting condition that would have happened regardless of the injury, and that the single trauma cannot be blamed for the individual's current problems, or he or she may claim that no scientific study has ever "proven" that trauma causes fibromyalgia.

Even though well-informed physicians should know and recognize fibromyalgia, many competent, credentialed and certified physicians will testify to the nonexistence of this condition, unfortunately.

Expert medical witnesses will be asked to provide opinions to a reasonable degree of medical certainty as to whether or not the individual has fibromyalgia and, if so, whether it was the trauma of the motor vehicle accident that caused this condition.

Even though we don't yet have studies that scientifically "prove" that trauma can cause fibromyalgia, we have strong clinical evidence that indicates that trauma causes fibromyalgia within medical and legal probability. One does not have to have scientific "proof" for all conditions we treat, just good clinical data. Most conditions we treat do not have the "scientific proof" studies, but that doesn't mean the condition doesn't exist or can't be treated. Medical definitions and legal definitions may differ, but the doctor tries to treat based on the clinical and medical information.

In the worker's realm, posttraumatic fibromyalgia can occur either from a single severe injury or as the result of accumulation of minor traumas, otherwise known as cumulative trauma. Once posttraumatic fibromyalgia is diagnosed, it becomes the "allowed condition," which indicates that the Worker's Compensation system recognizes that a certain job injury caused fibromyalgia. Any functional impairment due to this medical problem is determined, and this information can be used to ultimately determine any permanent or partial disability.

My philosophy is that fibromyalgia should never be truly totally and permanently disabling despite the functional impairment that it may cause. I try to help each patient achieve the highest of abilities despite the fibromyalgia. Each patient, however, has an individual set of circumstances that needs to be closely examined. At times a person may have such severe fibromyalgia that doesn't respond to treatment, that he or she is rendered totally disabled.

The Americans with Disability Act recently went into effect, otherwise known as ADA. ADA was designed to limit job discrimination against people

> Posttraumatic fibromyalgia can occur either from a single severe injury or as the result of accumulation of minor traumas, otherwise known as cumulative trauma.

> Since fibromyalgia can cause varying degrees of disability, this condition technically falls under the realm of... [the] Americans with Disability Act ...

who have disabilities. Since fibromyalgia can cause varying degrees of disability, this condition technically falls under the realm of ADA as it relates to the workplace.

ADA says that a qualified individual with a disability who can perform the essential functions of his job cannot be discriminated against. The employer is required to make reasonable accommodations for this qualified individual unless it would impose undue hardship. Reasonable accommodation and undue hardship are not clearly defined, unfortunately, under ADA.

If fibromyalgia is impairing one's ability to perform an essential job function, the employer is required, at the very least, to investigate the possibility of making a change at the job site to accommodate this individual. Under the spirit of the law, the employer should try to accommodate the individual with fibromyalgia by modifying the job duties so they are within this person's functional restrictions, or by supplying adaptive devices, such as an ergonomic chair, if these changes will allow the individual to continue the job successfully.

This new law is still being carefully analyzed by both sides, and we need to wait to see the full impact of this law, especially as it relates to fibromyalgia. If you have specific questions regarding your individual situation at the workplace, you should seek advice from the ADA experts.

This chapter is for your information and is not meant to be legal advice. You need to seek proper legal counsel from a qualified attorney if you have specific legal questions regarding fibromyalgia.

Fibromyalgia is a chronic and permanent condition. Painful tender points can become latent over time, but the overall condition does not disappear. The natural course is characterized by chronic pain and periodic exacerbations or flare-ups especially when the person is exposed to the specific risk factors or modulating factors that have been described.

It appears that over time about a third of people with fibromyalgia will have a stable course that does not get any better or any worse, but consistently flares-up; a third of the people will have improvement even though the condition doesn't disappear, and a third of the people will get worse. Therefore, any given individual with fibromyalgia may have a better than 50% chance that his or her condition will either stay the same or improve over the course of time.

There is no way of predicting what course any individual's fibromyalgia will take over time. The condition can remain stable for years, quickly change, or do any number of combinations. There is no evidence that fibromyalgia syndrome converts to a disease.

I believe that individuals who develop a program to successfully deal with fibromyalgia will be able to successfully change the course of their fibromyalgia. That is, someone who takes active measures to control the condition will be less likely to worsen over time due to the positive changes imparted upon the condition by working hard to improve health and well-being. The individual who does nothing to treat the fibromyalgia will probably have a higher risk of worsening over time.

My ongoing clinical experience supports that most people with fibromyalgia can do very well with their programs. I believe that our hard efforts in dealing with this condition will be rewarded in the long run by our feeling better and improving our overall condition.

29

Prognosis in Fibromyalgia

"Make the best use of what is in your power, and take the rest as it happens."

– Epictetus

Much research is being carried out to help us get a clearer picture of the fibromyalgia syndrome. Various research areas include:

1. Determining who is prone to getting this condition.

2. Researching the tender points, sympathetic nervous system, and biochemical pathways, to attempt to better understand the actual pathologic mechanism.

3. Studying individuals with this condition over time to determine what happens in response to long term treatments, and whether other conditions develop.

4. Studying the relationship between trauma, infection, and other factors that can cause fibromyalgia.

5. Developing new medications that are more selective and specific for controlling the neurotransmitters.

6. Identifying subgroups of the condition and studying regional versus general fibromyalgia.

Physicians of all specialties are learning more about fibromyalgia and are becoming better at diagnosing this condition. Industries and courts are also recognizing and understanding this condition better especially as it applies to social, economic and legal considerations.

The challenge is not only to fully understand fibromyalgia, but also to be able to minimize its impact on the individual and the community until a cure is found.

30

The Future and Fibromyalgia

"There is no medicine like hope, no incentive so great, and no tonic too powerful as expectation of something tomorrow."

– O. S. Marden

A

B

C

H

I

J

K

L

M

R

S

T

More Ways for "Helping You Live Life to the Fullest"

If you enjoyed *Fibromyalgia – Managing the Pain*, you will be interested in other resources from Anadem Publishing. Anadem Publishing is devoted to providing health information to assist patients with chronic conditions in taking charge of their recovery and in getting the most out of life.

The Fibromyalgia Survivor
by Mark J. Pellegrino, M.D.

The *Fibromyalgia Survivor* is packed with good advice and tips on every aspect of living your life to the fullest. You get the specific step-by-step "how to's" for daily living. Plus, you learn Fibronomics, the four key principles that help you minimize your pain in every situation.

The Fibromyalgia Supporter
by Mark J. Pellegrino, M.D.

How do you help loved ones really understand what they need to know about your fibromyalgia? Dr. Pellegrino explains to your loved ones how it feels, how they can become "supporters," and how you and your loved ones can still have a wonderful life together.

Understanding Post-Traumatic Fibromyalgia
by Mark J. Pellegrino, M.D.

Everyone with post-traumatic fibromyalgia will benefit from reading the first book focusing exclusively on this condition.

Laugh at Your Muscles
by Mark J. Pellegrino, M.D.

An easy, light read that you can enjoy and benefit from.

Chronic Fatigue Syndrome: Charting Your Course to Recovery
by Mary E. O'Brien, M.D.

Mary O'Brien, M.D., shares her personal experience in overcoming many of the debilitating effects of Chronic Fatigue Syndrome. In an easy-to-read, nontechnical format, Dr. O'Brien shares advice on treatment options and self-help steps that will help you rebuild your stamina.

TMJ – Its Many Faces
by Wesley Shankland, D.D.S., M.S.

Fibromyalgia patients frequently suffer from TMJ disorders and orofacial pain. Dr. Shankland's book is filled with step-by-step instructions on how to relieve TMJ, head, neck, and facial pain.

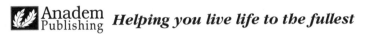 Anadem Publishing *Helping you live life to the fullest*

Order Your Books Today!

30 Day Money Back Guarantee
For fastest service, call 1•(800)•633•0055

Qty	Title	Price (US$)	Ohio Price*	Total
	Fibromyalgia:Managing the Pain	$12.45	$13.17	
	The Fibromyalgia Survivor	$19.50	$20.62	
	Understanding Post-Traumatic Fibromyalgia	$16.25	$17.18	
	The Fibromyalgia Supporter	$15.50	$16.39	
	TMJ – Its Many Faces	$19.50	$20.62	
	Laugh At Your Muscles	$ 5.95	$ 6.29	
	CFS – Charting Your Course to Recovery	$14.25	$15.07	

Shipping and handling

For 1 book, add $3.50
2–4 books, add $7.00
5–6 books, add $10.00
7+, please call
Priority mail, add $2.50

*Ohio price includes 5.75% state sales tax

Subtotal

➤ Add shipping and handling (see chart at left)

TOTAL

❑ Enclosed is my check, made payable to Anadem, Inc.
❑ Charge my credit card: ❑ 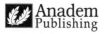 MasterCard ❑ VISA

Card No. _____ Exp. _____

Signature _____

Name _____

Address _____

City _____ State ____ Zip _____ Phone ( ) _____

Anadem Publishing   3620 North High Street • Columbus, OH • 43214
1-800-633-0055 • FAX (614) 262-6630
http://www.anadem.com

You can count on Anadem Publishing to keep you informed of the newest, most advanced ideas to help you get most out of life. Let us know if you want to be placed on our mailing list to be notified of new resources. And come visit us at our website! http://www.anadem.com